The Unspoken Grief of Men

A Companion Guide for Grieving Men from the Loss of a Loved One

S L Hans

Table of Contents

INTRODUCTION 1

CHAPTER 1: NAVIGATING THE LOSS OF A LOVED ONE 3

    THE CHALLENGE OF GRIEF...4

    TYPES OF LOSSES 6

        Spouse or Romantic Partner 6

        Child..7

        Parent 8

        Sibling or Close Friend..8

    COMMON FEELINGS ASSOCIATED WITH LOSS 9

    IMPORTANCE OF RECOGNIZING EMOTIONS..12

CHAPTER 2: UNDERSTANDING GRIEF 15

    THE MANY FACES OF GRIEF...15

    DISENFRANCHISED GRIEF: WHEN YOUR LOSS ISN'T RECOGNIZED..................16

    THE SPIRAL OF GRIEF 18

    THE PHYSIOLOGY OF GRIEF AND ITS IMPACT ON THE BODY 20

    HOW GRIEF REWIRES THE BRAIN 21

CHAPTER 3: THE EMOTIONAL ROLLERCOASTER 25

    THE SHOCK AND DISBELIEF OF EARLY GRIEF 26

    THE ANGER OF ANGUISH 27

    THE PIT OF DESPAIR AND DEPRESSION..29

    GUILT, REGRET, AND THINGS LEFT UNSAID 30

    LONELINESS IN THE AFTERMATH OF LOSS 31

    ANXIETY ABOUT AN UNCERTAIN FUTURE 32

    WHEN GRIEF GETS COMPLICATED 34

CHAPTER 4: GRIEF AND YOUR RELATIONSHIPS...37

    HOW GRIEF IMPACTS ROMANTIC RELATIONSHIPS 37

    THE CHANGING DYNAMICS OF FRIENDSHIPS AFTER LOSS............................38

    INTERACTING WITH COWORKERS WHILE GRIEVING 40

    DEALING WITH INSENSITIVE REACTIONS FROM OTHERS 42

    THE "EMPATHY SHORTCUT" FOR CONNECTING DESPITE GRIEF 44

CHAPTER 5: GRIEF AND YOUR IDENTITY **47**

GRIEF'S ASSAULT ON YOUR SENSE OF SELF.. 47

MASCULINITY AND THE PRESSURE TO "BE STRONG"............................... 48

FINDING YOURSELF AGAIN AFTER LOSS 50

POST-TRAUMATIC GROWTH: HOW GRIEF CAN CHANGE YOU FOR THE BETTER 51

CHAPTER 6: HEALTHY COPING STRATEGIES **55**

THE IMPORTANCE OF ACCEPTING YOUR FEELINGS AND CONSTRUCTIVE WAYS TO RELEASE
ANGER AND FRUSTRATION 55

HOW TO LET YOURSELF CRY 57

THE HEALING IMPORTANCE OF REMEMBRANCE AND RITUAL........................ 57

GRIEF JOURNALING FOR CLARITY AND CATHARSIS 58

MAKING SELF-CARE A PRIORITY 59

NUTRITION AND EXERCISE HELPS WITH GRIEF 60

SLEEP STRATEGIES AND ROUTINES AS ANCHORS 60

STAYING CONNECTED TO AVOID ISOLATION AND DISCOVERING NEW PURPOSE 61

CHAPTER 7: THE IMPORTANCE OF PROCESSING YOUR LOSS............................**63**

TELLING THE STORY OF YOUR LOVED ONE AND THE IMPORTANCE OF FACING PAIN 63

CONTINUING BONDS: REDEFINING YOUR RELATIONSHIP 65

COPING WITH BIRTHDAYS, HOLIDAYS AND ANNIVERSARIES 66

DEALING WITH YOUR LOVED ONE'S BELONGINGS 67

VISITING SPECIAL PLACES OF REMEMBRANCE.. 68

THE "GRIEF RELEASE" METHOD FOR LETTING GO...................................... 69

FINDING PEACE AND ACCEPTANCE 69

CHAPTER 8: FEELING STUCK **71**

MYTHS AND MISCONCEPTIONS ABOUT GRIEF 71

WHAT TO DO WHEN GRIEF FEELS UNBEARABLE 72

AVOIDING UNHEALTHY COPING MECHANISMS.. 73

OVERCOMING GUILT AND SELF-BLAME 74

BREAKING FREE FROM RUMINATION.. 75

COMBATING CHRONIC LONELINESS.. 76

CHAPTER 9: GRIEF AS A LIFELONG JOURNEY.................................**79**

WHY YOU WILL NEVER "GET OVER" YOUR LOSS 79

DEALING WITH GRIEF BURSTS AND SUDDEN SADNESS................................ 80

FINDING JOY AND ALLOWING YOURSELF TO LAUGH AGAIN 81

NEW RELATIONSHIPS AFTER LOSS 82

RELEARNING YOUR WORLD AS A GRIEVER 83

THE EVOLVING SEASONS OF GRIEF 85

HELPING OTHERS WITH YOUR HARD-WON WISDOM 86

CHAPTER 10: HONORING YOUR JOURNEY 89

UNDERSTANDING YOUR GRIEF JOURNEY 89

ACCEPTANCE AND ACKNOWLEDGEMENT 90

HONORING YOUR LOVED ONE AND YOURSELF 91

CONCLUSION 93

A NOTE FROM THE AUTHOR 95

REFERENCES 97

Introduction

I will not say: do not weep; for not all tears are an evil.
–J.R.R. Tolkien

Grieving the loss of a loved one is one of the most profound challenges of life, and if you are here, you are likely dealing with that very heartache. When it comes to men, most times we are expected to take care of our burdens silently and be the strong and steady pillar for others. Such expectations can make the process of grieving more painful and isolating. I have been there, and that is why I understand the struggle of dealing with grief alone. This book is for you—men who have lost someone close and those who support them.

You can regard this book as a companion to help you handle the unspoken grief that our culture or society wants us to hide. You might wonder what made me write this book. Well, it is because I have spent many years studying and understanding the unique ways in which men experience and express grief. Societal norms often tend to dictate that men are required to stay composed and apathetic. However, what we fail to understand is that this can suppress the natural process of grieving. This book explores such societal expectations and the differences in how men and women grieve, providing you with practical advice and insights to help you heal.

Losing someone you love and care for is never an easy thing, whether it takes place unexpectedly or slowly over time. If you have lost a loved one suddenly, you might feel like the ground has been pulled from under you without any warning. There is no time to say the last goodbye, or even be mentally prepared, and this shock can be crushing to the soul. It is a sudden emotional storm that can make you feel disoriented and lost. On the other hand, an anticipated loss, which might seem more manageable, comes with its own weight of stress. Knowing that a loved one is on the tail end of life's journey can bring prolonged anxiety and worry, just like a constant shadow that looms over your days. You are most likely to find yourself on an emotional rollercoaster, battling grief even before the actual loss takes place. Such a kind of grief might turn out to be even more intense, coupled with the stress of watching someone you love suffer.

Both kinds of losses are painful in their respective ways. There are various studies that have shown how such experiences might affect us differently. For instance, according to "Grief, Bereavement, and Coping With Loss" by the National Cancer Institute, sudden loss can result in acute stress reactions coupled with a sense of disbelief. On the other hand, anticipated loss might lead to emotional exhaustion and chronic stress (Grief, Bereavement, and Coping with Loss, 2017). Having a clear understanding of such differences can provide you with the requisite help to take care of your own grieving process in a compassionate way. Men always face societal expectations to be steady and strong, which can hamper the overall expression of pain. This might result in feelings of isolation, along with a lack of support, during the most vulnerable times of life.

It is necessary to understand that grieving might not look the same for everyone. And that is completely okay. I am here with this book to help you validate your feelings and provide a proper roadmap that can help you go through the complicated terrain of loss. Whether you are trying to cope with the immediate shock of a sudden loss or the long sorrow of an anticipated one, my primary objective is to provide you with a helping hand and make you understand that your feelings are valid and that there is no "correct" way to grieve. My journey has taught me that grieving cannot be regarded as a sign of weakness. If anything, it is a testament to the love we carry for the people who are no longer with us. Simply by addressing the unspoken grief of men, it is possible to break down all the hurdles that tend to delay healing and develop a compassionate place for ourselves and other people. Keep in mind that it is not at all about being a "strong" individual all the time. It is about being able to find the required strength in understanding and processing your pain. I hope this book can help you find a way forward.

Chapter 1:
Navigating the Loss of a Loved One

Grief is the price we pay for love.
–Queen Elizabeth II

Trying to navigate the loss of a loved one is one of the most challenging of life's experiences. In this section, we will explore the complex journey of grief, right from the initial shock to the long-term or sometimes never-ending process of healing. Before we begin this chapter, I would like to share the story of my close friend Nicholas, who lost his father unexpectedly. Nicholas was the kind of guy that everyone used to depend on, the first name which came to mind whenever there was something related to support and strength. When he lost his mother, he felt an overwhelming sense of confusion and loss. In fact, he was not even able to express his emotions, feeling the pressure to stay composed in front of his family. Nicholas disclosed to me about the nights when he used to stay awake, trying to take care of his grief single-handedly, as he never wanted to burden others with the pain he felt.

It can be said that what Nicholas experienced is not unique. There are several men who find themselves in such situations, not having any idea regarding how their feelings can be dealt with. The primary aim of this chapter is to provide you with the understanding that it is completely okay to grieve and seek help. By sharing stories like Nicholas's and with some practical advice, I hope to provide you with the right kind of guidance through such difficult times with support and empathy. Remember what C.S. Lewis said: "Grief is like a long valley, a winding valley where any bend may reveal a totally new landscape". (*A Quote from a Grief Observed*, n.d.)

The Challenge of Grief

Having a clear understanding of grief is crucial to navigating one of the most challenging journeys of life. Grief can never be regarded as a one-size-fits-all kind of experience. It is extremely unique and personal for everyone in this world. When you lose someone you love, the pain can turn out to be overwhelming, and the overall process of grieving might take various forms. But what is grief? It is a natural response to loss, which encompasses a wide range of thoughts, behaviors, and emotions. It is not only about feeling sad but could also encompass feelings of confusion, guilt, and anger based on the circumstances of the loss. For some, grief might seem like a tidal wave of emotions that comes crashing down all at once. For others, it might be an ongoing and slow process that might increase or decrease with time.

As men, we often tend to face new kinds of challenges when it comes to dealing with grief. The society of today, shaped by norms and popular culture - movies, art, music, and even funeral rites – typically expects us to be the pillars of strength, the ones who can hold things together when everything else seems to be falling apart. Such an expectation can make it hard for us to express our emotions or feelings in the right way. In fact, we might experience pressure to suppress our grief, maintain a stiff upper lip, and keep moving on in life as if nothing has changed. However, the truth is that our lives just turn upside down the moment we lose someone close. What we fail to understand is that trying to suppress grief can lead to serious consequences. It might result in feelings of depression, isolation, and even physical health issues. Acknowledging and expressing grief is never a sign of weakness; it is an important part of the healing process.

It has been found that men and women tend to cope with grief in different ways. It is said that men are more likely to engage in "instrumental" grieving. This means men might focus on problem-solving tasks, take on new duties or responsibilities, or keep themselves engaged in work as a way of taking care of their emotions. On the other hand, women are more likely to engage in "intuitive" grieving, which often involves an open expression of emotions, followed by the seeking of social support (Understanding Different Grieving Patterns in Your Family, 2017). Such differences might not be absolute, but they can help us understand why men might find it difficult to express their grief openly. We often feel more comfortable doing something tangible to honor our loved ones or work towards regaining a sense of control. However, it is also necessary to find ways in which you can connect with your emotions and seek support when you require it the most.

Perhaps one of the most challenging aspects of grief is its unpredictability. You might find yourself completely okay one moment, only to get hit by a sudden wave of sadness the next. I can assure you that this is normal. When it comes to grief, there is no linear path. It is like a winding road which has several ups and downs. Keep in mind that it is extremely crucial to be patient with yourself and to let yourself feel the emotions that arise. Looking back on my journey through grief, I found that talking to other people who experienced similar losses was extremely helpful. Hearing others and sharing your story can help in the creation of a sense of understanding and connection. It can remind you that you are not alone in your pain and that there are other people who have also walked this path. Professional support might turn out to be invaluable. Grief therapists and counselors are trained to help you navigate the complexity of loss. They can provide you with a safe space where you can express your emotions, offer practical strategies for coping, and help you figure out your way ahead.

Another often overlooked aspect of grief is the kind of physical impact it can have. Grief can take a serious toll on your body, resulting in symptoms like changes in appetite, fatigue, and problems falling asleep. Taking care of your physical health is an essential part of the grieving process. You will have to make sure that you get enough rest, eat well, and take part in physical activities that you actually enjoy. Finding ways to honor and remember your loved one can be a meaningful part of your healing journey. This might involve taking part in activities that were important to them, creating a memorial, or something as simple as taking time to reflect on your memories together. Such simple acts can help provide a sense of connection and continuity, providing you with all the help you need to keep their memory alive in your heart.

It is equally important to allow yourself to experience joy again and to keep living your life. At times, grief can make you feel guilty for moving ahead or for feeling happy, but it is important to keep in mind that the person you lost will always want you to find fulfillment and peace. Let yourself experience the full range of emotions that come with your everyday life, and know that it is absolutely okay to find happiness once again. Your grieving and healing journey will be as unique as your connection with the person you have lost. I would suggest you be gentle with yourself, get support or help whenever required, and have faith that, with time, the intensity of your pain will subside. Grief is a testament to the love you have for the person who is no longer with you or by your side. It is a process that will take time, but with the right kind of support and patience, you can find a way to heal and honor their memory.

Types of Losses

Losing someone who is close to you can never be regarded as an easy thing, and each kind of loss comes with its own set of emotions and challenges. Whether it is a spouse, a parent, a child, or a sibling, the pain is profound and deeply personal. I have been through my own experiences of grief and have talked to several men who have faced such heartbreaking losses. In this section, we will talk about the different types of losses and share some real-life stories with you so that you can also learn how to navigate the difficult journeys of life.

Spouse or Romantic Partner

Losing a romantic partner or spouse can be one of the most devastating experiences that a person can face. The individual you shared your life with, your daily routines, and your hopes, dreams, and aspirations are gone suddenly, leaving behind a huge void that might not seem possible to fill. The grief is not only for the person who is no more but also for the future days that you thought of together. I remember talking to Michael, a close friend who lost someone he regarded as his soulmate, Sandra, to cancer. They had been married for 15 years, and the bond they shared was extremely strong. When Sandra passed away, Michael felt lost. It can be said that his world turned upside down. He struggled with the sudden silence in their home and the lack of Sandra's presence in everything: the empty side of the bed, the absence of her laughter, the sounds of her making coffee in the kitchen, and their weekly movie night out together.

Initially, Michael made himself busy with his work so that he could avoid the pain - one of the most common responses among men. However, with time, he got to understand that it was not possible to run away from his grief. He started to take part in a support group for widowers, where he found peace as he shared his feelings with other men who actually understood the pain he had been experiencing. Michael also started to see a therapist, who provided him with a helping hand to process his emotions and figure out ways to remember Sandra while rebuilding his life again. The journey was not at all easy, but with time, Michael found a new normal and learned how he could live with his loss.

Child

The loss of a child is a pain that cannot be described in words. It is something that cuts to the core of one's being. It is a kind of grief that feels unfair and unnatural. The dreams that you had for the future of your child get shattered suddenly, and the emptiness they leave behind is immense. A friend of mine, Trevor, experienced this heartbreaking loss when his teenage son, Alex, died in a car accident. Trevor was engulfed by a mix of guilt, anger, and profound sadness. He started to feel that he had failed as a father, even though there was nothing he could have done to prevent the accident. The sudden loss tested every part of his being, including his connection with his wife. In fact, he seemed to have lost his sense of identity.

Luckily, Trevor found some comfort as he started connecting with other fathers who had lost their children. He attended a bereavement group where he could share his pain openly without any fear of being judged. Trevor also started a scholarship fund in the name of his son, which provided him with a way to honor his son's memory and keep his legacy alive. It is true that the pain might never fully go away, but it is with the help of such actions that Trevor found a way to channel his grief into something meaningful and positive.

Parent

Losing a parent, even as an adult, is one of the most significant and deep emotional experiences. Our parents are our first connection to the world, and their sudden death might bring about a sense of losing a major part of our history and foundation. Jason, an old friend of mine, lost his mother after a long battle with Alzheimer's disease. Jason spent most of his life watching the slow decline of his mother, feeling a mix of grief and relief as she passed away. The long illness gave him the necessary time to prepare, but the finality of death still hit hard. Jason struggled a lot with the sudden shift from being a caregiver to dealing with his own grief.

Jason's way of coping involved getting indulged in the past of his mother. He started sorting through old photos, family mementos, and letters, bringing together memories and stories that he wasn't aware of before. This process helped him feel connected to his mother in a completely new way and provided necessary comfort during the difficult early months of mourning. He also made a point of sharing such stories with his own children, making sure that the legacy of his mother would continue.

Sibling or Close Friend

The loss of a close friend or sibling often gets overlooked. However, it is a grief that is felt deeply. Close friends and siblings are the companions of our lives—the ones who share our history and actually understand us in ways others might not. Drake, a colleague of mine, lost his younger brother, Markus, to a sudden heart attack. Markus was only 30, and his sudden demise came as a shock to everybody. Drake found himself filled with a sense of anger and disbelief. He missed the inside jokes only they shared, their late-night conversations, and the millions of plans they had for the future.

Drake's grief journey involved reaching out to Markus' friends and other family members. They would gather to share stories and remember Markus, which helped Drake a lot - to feel less alone in his grief. In fact, he took up running, something that was loved by Markus, as a way to feel closer to his brother and to process his emotions. It was with the help of such activities that Drake found a way to honor the memory of his late brother and deal with the deep sense of loss.

It is necessary to find what works for you, whether it is engaging in activities that bring you comfort, seeking support from others, or finding ways to honor and remember the person you lost.

Common Feelings Associated With Loss

Experiencing the loss of a loved one is a personal journey, and it often starts with a whirlwind of emotions that might seem overwhelming. I will share some common feelings associated with loss. I can reassure you that such reactions are completely normal. If you find it hard to understand or cope with the emotions you feel, know that you are not alone. There are many others like you who have walked this path and experienced the same kinds of feelings.

- **Shock:** Shock is often the very first emotion that might hit you when you lose someone close. It might feel like a numbing sensation, as if you are trying to go through life in a dense fog. It is an initial disbelief that might act like a temporary buffer, letting you process the reality of the loss. It is the way in which your mind protects you from the overall impact of the grief at once. As you slowly come to terms with all that has happened, this sense of shock is most likely to fade away. However, it might resurface unexpectedly, specifically during moments that tend to remind you of your loved one.

- **Anger:** Anger is another common emotion that most men experience after a loss. You might find yourself feeling angry at the situation, at the individual who has left you, at other people who simply cannot understand your pain, and even at yourself.

Such anger mostly stems from a sense of frustration or injustice at the circumstances of the loss. It is necessary to acknowledge all feelings instead of trying to suppress them. Remember that anger can turn out to be a powerful force that can be constructive if you permit yourself to re-channel it in healthy ways: through talking it out, engaging in physical activity, or funneling the energy into something creative.

- **Guilt:** Guilt is an emotion that often accompanies grief, manifesting as thoughts of "if only" or "what if". Due to this, you might replay moments leading up to the loss, constantly questioning whether there was something that you could have done to stop it from happening. Guilt might also emerge from surviving, feeling like you should have been the one to die instead of your loved one, or simply feeling like you did not do enough for them while they were alive. It is important to make yourself understand that it is not possible to control or predict everything. Be gentle with yourself and remind yourself that it is normal to have such thoughts, but they must never define your reality.

- **Sadness:** Sadness can be regarded as the most common emotion while going through loss. The sorrow of missing someone who has been an integral part of your life might seem like a never-ending well of heartache and tears. It is okay to feel this sadness and allow yourself to cry it out. Tears are a natural way for the body to release all kinds of intense emotions that tend to build up. Let yourself grieve openly. There is nothing to be ashamed of. Crying is a crucial part of healing, and it's okay to cry.

- **Confusion:** An emotion that might catch you off-guard is confusion. When you lose someone, this might alter your sense of normalcy and hamper your everyday routine. You might most likely feel disoriented, finding it hard to make decisions or to concentrate on tasks that once used to come easily. Such confusion is a natural part of adjusting to a new reality where you do not have your loved one by your side. Provide yourself time to find your footing again, and try not to be too hard on yourself when things take longer than usual to get back to normal.

- **Loneliness:** Loneliness can be quite acute when you lose someone close. The person you lost may have been your partner in crime, your confidant, or someone who really understood you. Their absence can leave a void that is most likely to make you feel isolated, even when you are surrounded by other people. It is crucial to reach out and connect with others who care about you. Sharing your feelings with family, friends, or support groups can help bridge the gap and make you understand that you are not alone.

- **Anxiety and fear:** Anxiety and fear are emotions common after a loss. You might start worrying about what the future holds without your loved one or about your ability to take care of the situation. The loss might trigger existential questions and fears about the safety of other loved ones or your own mortality. It is quite normal to feel this way. Trying to talk about your fears can help alleviate some of this anxiety.

- **Relief:** Although this emotion might seem contradictory, relief can also be a part of the grieving process, specifically if your loved one was suffering. It is necessary to understand that feeling relief does not indicate that you loved the person any less. It simply acknowledges that their suffering has ended. Let yourself accept this feeling without any kind of guilt. It is nothing more than a part of the complicated tapestry of emotions that grief weaves.

- **Emotional numbness:** Emotional numbness may set in at times, especially after the initial shock. You might find yourself completely detached from what is happening around you and feel no connection to your own emotions. Such kinds of involuntary numbness are a way of coping, providing your mind a break from the intensity of your feelings. As you slowly start to heal, such periods of numbness will be less frequent.

Physical symptoms are also common. You might experience changes in appetite, feel fatigued, or find difficulty sleeping. Your body is deeply connected to your emotional state, and grief might manifest in physical ways. It is crucial to take proper care of yourself during this time, even if it is small acts of self-care such as getting some fresh air, eating regularly, or taking rest whenever possible.

Grieving is a process that takes time, and there is no set timeline for when you can start to feel better. It is an unpredictable journey that comes with good and bad days. What is more important here is to let yourself experience your grief fully. It is alright to seek help if you need it. As you try to navigate through these emotions, make sure you are kind to yourself. While the pain of loss is evident, it is also a reminder of the depth of your love for your loved one. With time, the intensity of pain will lessen, and you will start to find moments of peace and joy again. It is a gradual process, and it is completely okay to take it one step at a time.

Importance of Recognizing Emotions

Recognizing and understanding your emotions is an important step in taking care of grief. At times, it might feel overwhelming, but trying to acknowledge what you might be feeling can directly impact your overall healing journey. Emotions at the time of grief are complicated and varied. However, understanding and accepting them is a key part of moving ahead in life. As you lose someone important, it is quite natural to experience a wide range of emotions, from anger and shock to guilt and sadness, as we have discussed in the last section. Such feelings are your body and mind's way of processing the loss and starting to heal. When you recognize such emotions, you let yourself confront and work through them instead of suppressing them, which might otherwise result in long-term emotional problems.

One of the most compelling reasons to recognize your emotions is tied to resilience, which is our ability to get back up from setbacks or difficult experiences. It has been found that people who acknowledge and express their emotions can adapt more effectively to the loss. Resilience is not about avoiding grief. It is about embracing it head-on and letting ourselves experience the full range of emotions that come along with it (Mancini & Bonanno, 2009). Suppressing or ignoring emotions might result in complicated grief, an intense and prolonged state of mourning that can easily affect your ability to function. When emotions fail to be acknowledged, they won't disappear. They might end up manifesting in various unhealthy ways, like depression, anxiety, or physical health problems. Being able to recognize your emotions can help in the prevention of all these by directly addressing the grief and determining ways to deal with it.

During my own experiences with loss, I found that my emotions could be a vital part of healing when I named and accepted them. No, it has nothing to do with rushing through grief or trying to "get over it" as soon as you can. It is about allowing yourself to feel emotions deeply and understand what they mean. For instance, acknowledging that what you feel is anger might help you realize that it is coming from a place of feeling powerless or being treated unfairly by the overall situation. Such a kind of realization is crucial, as it can give a clear picture of what you are actually going through. Once you identify your emotions, you can start addressing them in healthy ways. This might involve writing in a journal, talking to a therapist or friend, finding creative outlets, or engaging in physical activity. Another great benefit of recognizing your emotions is that it can help enhance your relationships. Grief is powerful enough to develop barriers between you and the people around you, especially when you fail to express what you feel. But when you acknowledge and communicate your emotions, it can help others understand what you are actually going through. This can help foster deeper connections and provide the kind of support you require.

Sharing your feelings of loneliness or sadness with a family member or a close friend can bring understanding and comfort. It is true that they might not have the perfect words to say, but their presence and eagerness to listen can turn out to be extremely supportive. In fact, it can help break down the societal expectation that men are required to be stoic and cannot showcase vulnerability. Embracing your emotions can pave the way for a more honest dialogue about grief, cutting down the stigma around the expression of feelings. Keep in mind that recognizing your emotions is also about self-compassion. It is one of the easiest things to be hard on yourself at a time of grief, to feel like you should be taking care of things better or that you are not that strong. You will have to understand that grief is not a test of strength. It is a natural response when you lose someone close. Being compassionate with yourself means accepting that it is okay to feel the way you are feeling.

It is also said that those who practice self-compassion during times of grief can cope better. When you treat yourself with the same kind of kindness and understanding that you would offer a friend, you can develop a nurturing environment for healing. Self-compassion also involves recognizing that suffering is a universal experience and that there are many others like you who are in pain. This perspective can help remove feelings of isolation and deliver a sense of support and connection. It is also necessary to note that recognizing emotions does not indicate that you will get overwhelmed by them. It is about determining a balance where you get to acknowledge what you feel without getting consumed by it. This might involve setting aside some time to grieve while also making sure that you take part in activities that bring you comfort and joy. It is about letting yourself feel sad and miss your loved one while also allowing yourself moments of peace and happiness.

It is time that we move on to the next phase of our journey: understanding grief in detail.

Chapter 2:
Understanding Grief

Only people who are capable of loving strongly can also suffer great sorrow,
but this same necessity of loving serves to counteract their grief and heals them.
–Leo Tolstoy

Grief is a journey that looks different for everyone, and it might often seem like one is trying to navigate uncharted waters. In this chapter, we will delve deeper into the world of grief. By gaining insight into the nature of grief and its nuances, you can better equip yourself to deal with the waves of emotions that come your way and find a way towards acceptance and resilience.

The Many Faces of Grief

It can be said that grief is a personal and often misunderstood journey. It might manifest in various forms, and recognizing the different faces can help you deal with the pain.

- **Normal or common grief:** This is the kind of grief that most individuals are familiar with. It is grief that follows the expected stages, where disbelief, shock, and denial mark the immediate aftermath of a loss. These are often followed by intense emotions and deep longing for the person you have lost. With time, although the pain might never disappear completely, it can be more manageable. Life starts to move ahead, and we simply learn to start living with the loss. It is said that the majority of people experience this type of grief, which tends to resolve in some way or another within a few years.

- **Anticipatory grief:** This is the sorrow we feel before the actual loss takes place. Anticipatory grief can be regarded as a kind of premature mourning that starts when we know a loved one is nearing the end. I can recall an interview with Henry, a mental health counselor, who shared his personal experience with this kind of grief. When his grandfather was diagnosed with Alzheimer's disease, he experienced a whirlwind of worry, exhaustion, and sadness as he watched his grandfather slowly slip away. Such a kind of grief can be quite challenging, as it combines the pain of losing a loved one with the burden of caregiving.

- **Complicated grief:** This kind of grief deviates from the expected process of mourning. It includes various subtypes: chronic grief, delayed grief, and absent grief. Chronic grief tends to persist longer compared to typical grief, which is often accompanied by symptoms of anxiety or depression. Delayed grief surfaces without any notice, at times months or years after losing a loved one. On the other hand, absent grief is generally characterized by a lack of visible mourning, which is often the result of deep avoidance or denial of the emotional pain.

- **Distorted grief:** Distorted grief often manifests in intense ways. For instance, you might exhibit depression or anger without feeling sadness or loss. There are people who are well aware of the clear reality but still believe that their deceased loved one will come back. Such a kind of denial often results in unreasonable expectations and strained connections with others, reflecting the complicated nature of this kind of grief.

Disenfranchised Grief: When Your Loss Isn't Recognized

We all know that grief is a complicated experience. However, one of the most challenging forms of grief to deal with is disenfranchised grief. This kind of grief was first discussed by Kenneth Doka in his seminal 1989 study, "Disenfranchised Grief: Recognizing Hidden Sorrow." It refers to a loss that is not recognized socially or openly acknowledged. It is the kind of grief that most people suffer in silence, as it is not considered by society as a "legitimate" loss, especially when it comes to men (Disenfranchised Grief, 2023).

Disenfranchised grief might occur in various kinds of situations, and it might also be influenced by societal expectations and norms. The society in which we live today tends to have a rigid idea regarding what types of losses are worthy of public mourning and support. For instance, losing a spouse or a family member gets recognized easily and evokes a strong support network. But other types of losses, like a miscarriage, the death of an ex-partner, or the loss of a friendship, often fail to get the same kind of recognition. This lack of acknowledgment might make the process of grieving more painful and isolating. I remember talking to Jasper, a coworker who experienced this kind of grief. Jasper had a close relationship with his mentor, a man who was like a father to him throughout his career. The sudden death of his mentor devastated Jasper. However, he came to find that the grief he experienced was not at all taken into serious consideration by people around him. His colleagues offered condolences but moved on quickly. In fact, his family failed to understand the depth of his sorrow. They failed to see the profound impact the loss had on his life, and Jasper felt like he had been shortchanged to grieve intensely for a person who was not a blood relative.

Jasper's experience is a classic example of what disenfranchising grief looks like. According to the study by Kenneth Doka (1989), grief of this kind is often marginalized as it fails to fit properly into the framework of loss that is accepted socially. Our society tends to create a hierarchy of grief, where certain connections are regarded as more important or significant compared to others. This same hierarchy dictates who can mourn openly and who cannot. Such a social framework can turn out to be specifically challenging for men, who are always expected to be strong and unemotional. Men who face disenfranchised grief might experience additional pressure to suppress their emotions. Traditional gender norms often discourage men from expressing vulnerability. This societal expectation might result in an internalized shame and a hesitancy to seek support. For Jasper, the combination of such factors made the grieving process extremely lonely. He always felt that he had to put on a brave face at work and also in front of his family, suppressing his true feelings inside himself and dealing with his loss in isolation.

It is necessary to understand that trying to deal with disenfranchised grief will require a great degree of resilience. It might also require a shift in perspective. For Jasper, finding a way to honor the memory of his mentor became an important part of his healing journey. He started to write down the lessons and stories he learned from his mentor. Doing so not only helped him process the grief but also helped preserve the legacy of his mentor. Jasper also went to other people who were close to his mentor and created a small community where they could share their memories openly. The story of Jasper illustrates the importance of finding support and validation, even at times when it is not available from society. Doka's research focuses on understanding that acknowledging disenfranchised grief is the first step toward addressing it. Simply by recognizing that such hidden sorrows are valid, it is possible to create spaces where all forms of loss are mourned and respected

If you are also experiencing disenfranchised grief, know that your feelings are completely legit. It is important that you find ways to express and validate your grief, whether with the help of talking to trusted friends, journaling, or seeking professional help. The key here is to give yourself permission to mourn, regardless of all kinds of societal expectations. What I have learned from talking to many men like Jasper is that every loss, no matter how society sees it, deserves recognition. By acknowledging disenfranchised grief, you can start to break down the myriad of barriers that tend to stop you from fully grieving and healing.

The Spiral of Grief

Grief is a lot more complicated than we think it is. It does not move in a straight line from one stage to the next. In fact, it is more like a spiral, where we keep revisiting experiences and feelings repeatedly, at times when we least expect it. I have seen this in my own life and also through the experiences of other people. The concept of spiraling through the stages of grief is something that has been described properly by Elisabeth Kübler-Ross's model of grief stages. But it is necessary to understand that such stages—denial, anger, bargaining, depression, and acceptance—are not like a checklist that needs to be completed (Rogers, 2022). They are like elements that we can cycle through several times. A study was conducted by Maciejewski and his colleagues in 2007, and their findings challenged the traditional view of Kübler-Ross's model. The study suggested that while such stages are present, they might not occur in a specific order. In fact, they might not be experienced by everyone in the same way. It was also highlighted that grief is more fluid in nature. People might find themselves revisiting various stages at different points, showcasing the nonlinear nature of emotions (Pk et al., 2007).

I recall talking to a man named Thomson, who lost his father to a heart attack. The grief journey of Thomson can perfectly illustrate the spiral concept. During the initial days, he was in denial. He could not believe that his father, who had always seemed to be so strong and fit, was gone. This denial acted as a protective mechanism, letting him process the shock gradually. After a few weeks, his denial shifted to anger. Thomson found himself irrationally angry at his father for not being able to take better care of himself and at the doctors for not detecting his heart problems earlier. This anger was merged with moments of bargaining, where Thomson would think of all the "what ifs"—what if his father had gone to the doctor sooner? What if Thomson had been more insistent on daily check-ups? This was followed by depression, introducing a profound sadness that would generally come in waves. Some days, he felt like he would drown in his grief, not able to find motivation or joy in anything. On other days, the sadness would lower a bit, only to come back and attack later.

The study by Maciejewski and his colleagues emphasizes that people do not progress through these stages in a set order. They often end up spiraling through them, revisiting different stages and emotions as they try to process their loss. The spiral nature of grief can be confusing and exhausting, as just when you feel you are moving ahead, a familiar emotional wave will pull you back. However, this is a natural part of the grieving process. With time, Thomson learned to accept that his grief was not at all something that was required to be "completed". It is something that needs to be managed. He found solace in discussing his father, sharing memories with family and friends, and even in therapy sessions where he was able to express his sadness and anger without getting judged. It can be said that the spiral approach to understanding grief can help us to be more compassionate with ourselves and other people as well. In my conversations with others who also experienced loss, the spiraling theme of grief was constant. Whether it is an anniversary that brings up sudden, intense emotions or a sudden memory that triggers a new wave of sadness, such moments are part of the ebb and flow of grieving.

The Physiology of Grief and Its Impact on the Body

Most of us think of grief as an emotional experience. However, it is more than that. It can take a toll on our physical health as well. When we experience intense emotions, our bodies tend to respond in ways that can be both overwhelming and surprising. I have seen the same in my own life and in the lives of those around me, and it is something that science has been exploring to understand better. A 2018 study delves into the connection between our physical health and emotions. It was found that suppressing negative emotions does not only impact our mental state; it can also affect our physical health (Ruan et al., 2019). When we tend to store our grief or try not to deal with it, we might feel that we are taking care of it, but our bodies might tell a completely different story.

One of the most common physical symptoms of grief is fatigue. We might not understand this, but the weight of sorrow can be physically exhausting. It is not only about feeling tired; it is a deep fatigue that can make even the simplest tasks feel impossible. All of these happen because grief is a form of stress, and when our bodies are under stress for a long period of time, it can easily deplete our energy reserves. Due to this, our bodies need to work overtime in order to process all kinds of intense emotions, leaving us feeling drained. Another frequent symptom is a loss of appetite. When you grieve, your body is most likely to go into a kind of shock, hampering your everyday routines, including eating. Stress and sadness can result in a diminished interest in food, and at times, it might be difficult to collect the energy to consume food. This can collectively result in weight loss and nutritional issues, which further contribute to the feeling of weakness and exhaustion.

Sleep disturbances are quite common. Many grieving people tend to experience insomnia or restless sleep. The mind often keeps racing with memories and thoughts, making it hard to relax so that one can fall asleep. Even when sleep does come, it might be disrupted by nightmares or dreams related to the loss, resulting in non-restorative and fragmented sleep. This lack of quality sleep compounds fatigue and can have serious effects on one's overall health. Suppressing intense emotions might exacerbate physical symptoms. When we do not let ourselves experience and express our grief fully, we might notice a sudden increase in such physical manifestations. The body will hold onto the stress, and this can result in more severe problems such as headaches, chronic pain, and cardiovascular issues. It is crucial to understand that our emotions are directly linked to our physical state and trying to ignore one can affect the other.

Being able to understand the physiology of grief is important, as it underscores the importance of addressing both the physical and emotional aspects of health during such hard times. It is necessary to listen to our bodies and recognize the symptoms as part of the grieving process instead of simply ignoring them. Self-care becomes extremely important during times of grief. This indicates not only letting yourself express and feel the emotions but also taking proactive steps to support your physical health. Try to maintain a balanced diet, even when you do not feel like eating. Small portions of nutritious food can help maintain your energy levels. Try to prioritize rest, even when sleep is elusive. Light activities such as yoga or walking can help in the management of stress and enhance your overall quality of sleep. Do not hesitate to opt for professional help if required. Grief counselors, therapists, and support groups can provide you with the space to express your emotions and learn useful strategies so that you can deal with the physical toll of grief. Grief is not only in your mind, but it is a full-body experience that needs comprehensive care.

How Grief Rewires the Brain

Grief is an experience that goes beyond emotions and touches every part of our being, and that includes our brain as well. When we lose a loved one, the brain undergoes various kinds of changes, and understanding such changes can help us navigate this hard time with a bit more self-compassion and insight. It can be said that grief actually rewires the brain. When we develop deep connections with others, such relationships get etched into our neural pathways. So, when someone close to you dies, your brain needs to reorganize itself to adapt to the new reality. This overall process is not only emotional but deeply physiological as well. One of the primary brain areas that gets affected by grief is the prefrontal cortex. It is the part of the brain that is responsible for complicated cognitive behavior, moderating social behavior, and decision-making. At the time of grief, the prefrontal cortex might turn out to be less active. This explains why we tend to find it hard to make decisions, focus, or even perform daily routine tasks. I have personally experienced this disconnected and foggy feeling, and it can turn out to be pretty frustrating, especially when you try to maintain some normality.

Another important part of the brain that is involved in grief is the limbic system, which includes the hippocampus and amygdala. The amygdala is the emotional center of the brain, and it lights up at times of sadness and stress. While grieving, the amygdala gets highly active, which might result in heightened emotions coupled with an overwhelming sense of fear or anxiety. Such a heightened state of alertness can make it hard to feel safe or relaxed, even in familiar environments. On the other hand, the hippocampus is linked with learning and memory. Grief can impact the hippocampus in a way that can make recalling memories, both new and old, quite challenging. You might start feeling that you can no longer rely on your memory, or you might forget simple things. This is all because the release of stress hormones during grief disrupts the ability of the hippocampus to function in the right way.

A study delves into such changes, focusing on how the reward system of the brain also gets affected by grief (Wolf, 2024). The VTA, or ventral tegmental area, and the nucleus accumbens, brain parts involved in reward and pleasure, show reduced activity. Such a reduction might result in anhedonia, a condition in which you might lose interest in activities that you once loved. This is the reason why socializing, hobbies, or even having your favorite food might not seem appealing anymore. Grief might also impact the default mode network (DMN) of the brain. It remains active when the mind is at rest and not focused on the external world. The DMN is linked to memories, self-referential thoughts, and emotions. At the time of grief, the DMN might get overactive, resulting in rumination and continuous thoughts about the person you lost. This might trap you in a thought cycle about what could have been done differently or simply replaying the same memories over and over again.

Understanding such brain changes can make it easier for you to be easy on yourself. Recognizing that the brain is undergoing a complicated reorganization process can help you understand why grief feels so consuming. Taking proper care of your brain during this time is important. Practices such as mindfulness and meditation can help calm the amygdala and cut down the stress response. Opting for physical exercise can help boost endorphin production, improve cognitive function, and improve mood. By understanding how grief can rewire the brain, it is possible to take steps to support our emotional and mental health. It is okay to grieve in your own way, but do not be too hard on yourself.

Chapter 3:
The Emotional Rollercoaster

Grief is like the ocean; it comes on waves ebbing and flowing. Sometimes the water is calm, and sometimes it is overwhelming. All we can do is learn to swim.
–Vicki Harrison

Grief is a multifaceted and intense experience that can leave us feeling like we are on an emotional rollercoaster. The aim of this chapter is to explore this kind of emotional turbulence, focusing on the ups and downs that accompany loss and why understanding such emotions is important for navigating through them. Grief can never be regarded as a linear process. It is more like a chaotic ride that tends to take us through a myriad of feelings, mostly when we least expect it. This rollercoaster can leave you feeling overwhelmed, making it tough to function in your everyday life. It is necessary to acknowledge and understand such emotions, as this is the primary step in the direction of healing. For instance, when John, a friend of mine, lost his wife to a serious illness, he was thrown into a whirlwind of emotions. He experienced various kinds of emotional and physical symptoms that made his daily life almost intolerable. He had difficulty sleeping, felt fatigued all the time, and lost his appetite. At work, he found it difficult to focus and found himself easily irritated by minor things. John's grief was extremely consuming, affecting each and every aspect of his life.

It wasn't until John took the help of a grief counselor that he started to understand the profound ways in which grief was affecting his mind and body. The counselor helped him see that the way he reacted was normal and that his grief was nothing but a reflection of the deep love he had for his life partner. This understanding obviously did not make the pain vanish, but it provided him with tools to deal with and a sense of proper direction in his overall healing process. As author Anne Lamott said, "You will lose someone you can't live without, and your heart will be badly broken, and the bad news is that you never completely get over the loss of your beloved. But this is also the good news. They live forever in your broken heart, which doesn't seal back up. And you come through. It's like having a broken leg that never heals perfectly—that still

hurts when the weather gets cold, but you learn to dance with the limp."
(*A Quote by Anne Lamott*, n.d.)

Analyzing the impact of grief on your body and mind can help you devise strategies to deal with the loss. This might involve practicing self-care techniques like meditation, exercise, or journaling, along with getting the help of others who can understand all that you are going through. By recognizing the emotional rollercoaster of grief, you can find effective ways to navigate through it, finding moments of resilience and peace along the way.

The Shock and Disbelief of Early Grief

When grief strikes, it hits hard, often with an intensity that almost feels surreal. The disbelief and shock that comes along with early grief can turn out to be overwhelming. It is as if the mind cannot fully grasp the reality of the loss. It is a common initial reaction. When you face the sudden absence of a loved one, the brain is most likely to go into a protective mode, protecting you from the full effect of the pain. This reaction is not only emotional but physiological as well. There is a study that focuses on the impact of bereavement because of sudden death and explores how people react when confronted with a sudden loss. The research shows that sudden death can result in more intense feelings of disbelief and shock in comparison to anticipated loss. Such a shock can hamper the cognitive process, making it difficult to accept the reality of the situation and often resulting in feelings of detachment or numbness.

I recall talking to Tylor, a man who experienced this firsthand when he lost his partner, Laura, in an accident. One moment, she was texting him about their dinner plans, and the next moment, she was gone. Tylor described those initial days as living in a dense fog. He had to contact their families, arrange the funeral, and handle paperwork, but nothing felt real. Deep down inside, he expected to wake up from this bad dream. Even after a few weeks, he found himself reaching for his phone to text Laura, only to get hit by the devastating reality that she was no longer in this world. Tylor's shock was primarily compounded by the abruptness of his partner's death. He had no time to prepare and no chance to say goodbye. This is quite a common scene in sudden bereavement. The unexpected nature of sudden losses can exacerbate the initial shock, making it harder for the brain to process the overall event.

It is crucial to understand that this state of disbelief and shock is a normal part of the grieving process. It is the way in which the brain tries to shield itself from the overwhelming pain of loss. This sort of initial numbness might last from a few days to several weeks, and it serves as a buffer, providing us time to slowly accept the reality of the situation. During this time, you might find yourself completely detached from reality, as if you are watching your life unfold from a distance. Simple tasks might seem hard, and you might struggle to remember or focus on things. All of these are your mind's way of dealing with the trauma. Tylor found that talking about what he was feeling, even when it did not make much sense, helped him start processing the loss. He joined a support group for people who had lost their loved ones suddenly. Hearing others share their experiences reassured him that he was not alone in his disbelief and shock. Such a sense of community provided him with all the help he needed to begin moving forward in life, even if just in minute steps.

Shock and disbelief are not signs that you are not handling your grief in the right way. They are nothing more than natural responses to a situation that you never imagined. Let yourself feel such emotions without any kind of judgment. Reach out to other people, whether family, friends, or support groups, and share your experience. At times, simply knowing that all you are going through is completely normal can provide a great deal of comfort. The key takeaway here is that feeling shocked or disbelieving after you lose someone close is normal. These feelings are part of the brain's coping mechanisms. Remember that the initial shock will eventually provide you with a clearer understanding of your grief. It is a gradual process, and it is okay if you seek help along the way.

The Anger of Anguish

Grief has a way of pulling out emotions that we might never have expected to feel so intensely. One of the most difficult and surprising emotions to manage is anger. Whenever we think of grief, we tend to focus on sadness. However, anger is a force of the grieving process that needs understanding and attention. Anger at the time of grief might manifest in several ways. It might be directed at the person who has died, at the world in general, or at oneself. This anger might feel guilt-inducing and distracting, especially when the world around us expects us to mourn in silence. It is necessary to acknowledge that anger is a natural response to loss that is rooted in the frustration and helplessness that come along with death. There is a study that focuses on how men and women experience and express anger differently at times of grief. According to the study, men are more likely to showcase outward expressions of anger, whereas women might internalize what they feel (Chaplin, 2018). This does not indicate that men tend to grieve less deeply or that their grief is less valid. All it shows is that personal tendencies and societal norms can shape the way in which grief manifests. Understanding such differences can help address and manage grief in a better way.

I remember a conversation I had with a friend named Mark, who lost his mother to a serious illness. Mark was a person who was always calm and collected. But right after the death of his mother, he found himself filled with rage. He was angry at the doctors for not being able to catch the signs earlier, at his mother for not taking proper care of her health, and also at himself for not being more insistent on regular check-ups. In fact, this anger impacted other areas of his life, which made him irritable at work and distant from his friends and family. The experience of Mark shows how anger might catch us off guard. He described himself as feeling like a ticking time bomb, all set to explode over minute things. The anger he showed was his way of dealing with the sense of loss and helplessness that he experienced. Mark started talking to a therapist and came to realize that his anger was part of his grief. It was not something that he should suppress or be ashamed of.

Now, this lays the foundation for an important point: understanding and accepting your anger while grieving is necessary. Suppressing it might result in further physical and emotional distress. You need to find healthy ways in which you can express and manage this anger. Whether through seeking professional help, talking to a friend, engaging in physical activities, or writing about what you feel. The key here is to let the anger out, but in a constructive way. The study also highlights that while men might be more likely to express anger openly, it is necessary for everyone, regardless of gender, to figure out their own way in which they can process their feelings. Keep in mind that anger in grief is not always about the immediate situation. It often tends to touch on deeper feelings of fear, injustice, and sadness. Understanding this will let you be more compassionate with yourself and other people who are grieving.

The Pit of Despair and Depression

The deep sorrow that follows a significant loss might often plunge us into what feels like a pit of despair and depression. It is a consuming and heavy feeling that can make even the easiest tasks seem impossible. Despair and depression after a loss are not only about feelings of sadness. It is a sense of hopelessness and emptiness that can hamper your physical and mental health. Trying to deal with depression at a time of grief will need a lot more than just "toughing it out." It is important to recognize when the normal sadness of grief has taken the form of something serious. Professional help is often necessary to go through such challenging terrain. Counselors and therapists who specialize in grief can provide great support, providing you with strategies to cope with all kinds of overwhelming emotions and helping you stay away from heading toward deeper depression.

Seeking professional help might seem daunting, specifically when depression tends to sap your motivation and energy. But remember that reaching out is an important step in the direction of healing. Therapy can provide you with a safe space where you can express what you feel without getting judged and process the complicated emotions that come along with grief. CBT, or cognitive behavioral therapy, for instance, can be extremely effective in taking care of depression. It can help you identify and alter patterns of negative thoughts, developing a balanced perspective. Another option is medication. It can be useful for all those who tend to struggle with chronic depression. Antidepressants can help stabilize mood, making it easier for you to engage in therapy or other kinds of self-care practices. You can consult with a psychiatrist to ensure that medication is the correct choice for you. If not, you can work with them to determine the most effective plan of treatment.

Apart from professional help, there are practical steps that you can opt for to manage depression during grief. Developing a daily routine, even a simple one, can provide you with a sense of control and normalcy. Exercise, even if you can go for a short walk, can help improve mood by boosting endorphins. Consuming nutritious food items, getting adequate sleep, and staying hydrated are important when it comes to maintaining your physical health, which in turn can directly impact your mental health. Mindfulness and relaxation techniques, like deep breathing exercises, meditation, and yoga, can help in the reduction of anxiety while also promoting a sense of calm. Such practices can encourage you to be present, helping you manage all sorts of overwhelming thoughts that often come with grief and depression. It is important to be patient with yourself during this time. Healing from such a deep loss is not a linear process. It is normal to have good days and bad days.

Guilt, Regret, and Things Left Unsaid

When we lose someone close to us, it can leave us fighting with overwhelming feelings of regret and guilt. Such emotions are like twin shadows, haunting our thoughts and making it impossible to find peace. Regret and guilt are common responses to loss, but they are distinct experiences. Trying to understand them can help navigate through such tough emotions. Guilt develops when you start believing that you have failed in some way or done something wrong. It is linked to a sense of responsibility and the feeling that you have violated your ethical standards or morals. Such an emotion generally comes with a strong sense or desire to make amends or fix everything that went wrong, even though that is impossible when it comes to losing a loved one. On the other hand, regret is more about desiring things to have turned out differently. It is the sadness and disappointment over decisions or missed opportunities that fail to go as planned. Unlike guilt, regret does not involve any sort of moral failing. It comes with a deep longing for an alternate outcome.

From a psychological point of view, guilt is linked to our sense of morality. It is an acknowledgment that we believe we have fallen short of our own standards. This might result in intense feelings of remorse and a requirement to rectify or apologize. Regret is more reflective in nature. It might also involve looking back and thinking, "What if?". Trying to figure out all those areas where things could have been a bit different. When you lose someone, such emotions can be extremely intense. You are most likely to find yourself replaying events, wishing you had done or said something differently, or constantly blaming yourself for not being there enough. This is a common reaction. One of the most effective ways to deal with regret and guilt is through therapy. With the help of a professional, you can easily untangle the complicated emotions and get guidance towards healthier ways of coping.

Self-forgiveness is extremely important during this time. Understanding that everyone makes mistakes and that most situations are not within your control can help you stay away from harsh self-judgment. Trying to accept your imperfections and understanding that you gave your best can be liberating. Expressing your emotions is an important step. Whether through art, words, or physical activity, finding a way to let out your feelings can help ease the weight of regret and guilt. Lastly, it is crucial to reevaluate your expectations of yourself. Feelings of regret and guilt mostly stem from unrealistic standards. Try to remind yourself that it is okay to be imperfect. Adjusting your expectations can help you get rid of some of the regret and guilt.

Loneliness in the Aftermath of Loss

Losing someone close can cause an overwhelming sense of loneliness. It is not only about the absence of that person's presence. It is the quiet emptiness that tends to fill your days and the empty space at the dinner table. Such a kind of loneliness can creep into every aspect of your being, making even the most usual places seem foreign. When my friend David lost his wife, Marium, he found himself in an empty world. They had been married for more than 20 years, and their lives were so intertwined that her absence left a hole in his life. David shared how the evenings were the hardest. The silence in their home, which once felt comforting, now felt oppressive. Even the simplest routines, like watching TV at night or making dinner, reminded him of her painful absence.

David's experience is a common one. Loneliness right after losing someone close can be profound. It is not only the physical presence that is missing but also the companionship and emotional support. Family and friends might come forward with their support initially, but with the passage of time, they get back to their routines, and the bereaved can feel isolated in their grief. One of the most important steps in dealing with loneliness is acknowledging it. It is necessary to understand that feeling lonely after a loss is a natural part of the grieving process. Staying busy can help, but it is not only about filling time. It is about finding meaningful activities that can help create a sense of connection and purpose. Being part of a support group can be useful. Such groups provide a space where you can freely share your feelings with other people who can truly understand all that you are going through.

Another way to cope with loneliness is by staying connected with friends and family. Reaching out can make a huge difference. Even if it is just a coffee date or a phone call, such interactions can provide necessary emotional support. David made a point to call his children more often and also arranged for weekly lunches with his brother. Such small steps helped him feel less isolated and more connected. Engaging in activities that you enjoy or trying out something new can help. Interests and hobbies can provide a distraction in addition to a sense of accomplishment. David opted for gardening, something Marium loved. Taking care of the plants and watching them grow gave him a sense of connection to his wife and a brand-new way to channel all his emotions. Volunteering can turn out to be a powerful antidote to loneliness. Providing help to others can provide you with a sense of fulfillment and help you develop new social connections.

Anxiety About an Uncertain Future

Losing someone you love can turn your world upside down. It can make everything feel uncertain. This uncertainty can breed anxiety regarding the future. When my friend James lost his job only a few months after he lost his father, he found himself engulfed by a sense of fear and dread. James was the pillar of strength in his family. Losing his father was a huge blow, but losing his job so soon afterward felt like the ground was pulled from under his feet. The stability he was once dependent on was gone, and he found himself facing an uncertain future without any idea regarding how to move ahead. He shared with me that he was anxious all the time, his mind racing with thoughts about what might happen next, lying awake at night. He was worried about his career prospects, his finances, and whether he could take care of his family.

Anxiety after a significant loss is a common experience. The future, which seemed predictable once, now seemed like a frightening unknown. Such anxiety might manifest in multiple ways, from physical symptoms such as shortness of breath or a racing heart to mental ones such as a sense of impending doom and persistent worry. It is a natural response to feeling like your life is out of control. It is true that what James experienced is not unique. There are many people who find themselves struggling with intense anxiety after a major change or loss. It is necessary to recognize that there are ways to manage it. Let's have a look at some tips that can help.

- **Mindfulness techniques:** Practicing mindfulness on a daily basis can be quite effective in the management of anxiety. Mindfulness involves staying present and fully engaged in the current situation. Techniques like progressive muscle relaxation, deep breathing exercises, and mindful meditation can help calm your mind and cut down on anxiety. Whenever you find your thoughts spiraling into worry regarding the future, try to ground yourself by concentrating on your breath or the sensations that you feel in your body.

- **Developing a routine:** Developing a daily routine can provide a sense of predictability and structure, which can feel soothing when other things in life feel uncertain. Set small and achievable goals for every day and stick to a daily schedule. Doing so can help you regain a sense of stability and control.

- **Limiting exposure to stressors:** Try to figure out and limit exposure to all those things that tend to exacerbate your anxiety. This could mean reducing the time you spend watching the news or scrolling through social media. Concentrate on activities that bring you relaxation and joy.

- **Connect with other people:** Reach out to family, friends, or support groups. Talking about your concerns and feelings with all those who care about you can provide relief and help you deal with your loneliness. At times, simply knowing that you have other people to listen to can make a huge difference.

- **Break down problems:** When you face a daunting situation, try to break it down into smaller and manageable parts. Try to focus on all that you can do today or in the next hour instead of getting overwhelmed by the overall challenge. Such an approach can make problems seem less daunting.

- **Positive visualization:** Try to spend a few minutes every day visualizing all kinds of positive outcomes. Think of yourself taking care of future challenges successfully, and imagine all the steps that you will take to get there. This can help cut down on the fear of the unknown and develop confidence in your capability to cope.

- **Educating yourself:** Sometimes, anxiety might stem from a lack of information. Try to educate yourself about your overall situation and possible future outcomes or scenarios. It is possible to reduce fear with the help of knowledge. It can help you make informed decisions about the next steps.

James found a new job, but it took effort and time to get there. On his journey, he learned to take care of his anxiety by incorporating some of the above-mentioned techniques into his daily life. It is necessary to understand that feeling anxious about the future is a natural response to change and loss.

When Grief Gets Complicated

Losing someone close to us can shake us to the core. While most people slowly find a way to deal with grief, some might experience what is known as complicated grief. This type of grief might feel like being trapped in a never-ending circle of longing and sorrow, making it harder to move ahead in life. Complicated grief occurs when the normal process of mourning gets stuck and lasts a lot longer than usual. Unlike typical grief, which generally eases over time, complicated grief is most likely to persist, resulting in intense emotional pain and preventing people from resuming their everyday lives. According to a study, symptoms of complicated grief include an inability to accept the loss, persistent yearning for the deceased, problems trusting other people, and a sense of meaninglessness or emptiness. Such feelings can turn out to be so overwhelming that they end up interfering with the ability of a person to function (Shear et al., 2005).

One of the men I know, Matthew, went through this painful experience. He lost his brother in an accident, and his world was completely changed. While his family and friends slowly started to heal, Matthew was stuck in time. Every day felt like a real struggle. He was not able to focus on his work, stayed away from all kinds of social activities, and lost joy in the hobbies that he used to love. The thought of his brother's absence consumed him, and he could not think of life without this continuous ache. The condition of Matthew is a classic example of complicated grief. The intense and persistent sorrow and longing he experienced prevented him from moving ahead in life. It wasn't until he sought help from a therapist specializing in grief that things started to change. He was introduced to a treatment that was designed specifically for complicated grief. It was a method that was supported by the above-mentioned study. It was known as CGT, or complicated grief treatment. It involves a combination of cognitive-behavioral techniques and interpersonal therapy. It concentrates on helping people accept the truth of their loss, process the emotions they feel, and rebuild their lives.

With the help of this therapy, Matthew was encouraged to talk about his brother and the circumstances that resulted in his death in a supportive and structured environment. He slowly learned to confront his painful feelings instead of trying to run away from them. One of the most useful techniques for Matthew was creating a memory book filled with stories and photos of his brother. This permitted him to honor the memory of his brother while also understanding that his own life had to continue. Matthew also engaged in activities that helped him slowly re-engage with the world around him. His therapist provided him with a helping hand to set achievable and small goals, like meeting a friend for coffee or going for a walk every day. Such steps helped Matthew rebuild a sense of normalcy and find moments of joy amidst all the grief. It is true that the process was not that easy, and there were days when Matthew felt like he was going back to square one. But with the help of CGT and his therapist, he started to see changes. Complicated grief is an isolating and painful experience, but it is important to understand that it is treatable.

All kinds of intense emotions are natural parts of the grieving process. You will have to acknowledge them, understand them, and try to deal with them in ways that actually work for you without trying to suppress them.

Chapter 4:
Grief and Your Relationships

Sometimes, only one person is missing, and the whole world seems depopulated.
–Alphonse de Lamartine

Losing someone dear to us can affect every corner of our lives, and our relationships are no exception. In this chapter, we will explore how grief can reshape the dynamics of our connections with other people. When we deal with profound loss, we may notice that our interactions with family, friends, and colleagues change in unexpected ways. Whether it is your romantic relationship, your role as a parent, or your friendships, grief can change the way in which you relate to people around you. Recognizing how grief affects your relationships can provide support and insight as you try to work through this challenging time.

How Grief Impacts Romantic Relationships

When you lose someone important to you, it is not just your own heart that breaks. Your romantic relationship might also face a huge strain. In the aftermath of a loss, how you and your partner experience and express grief might differ to a huge extent. Such differences can result in misunderstandings, frustration, and a sense of emotional gap that might turn out to be a hard thing to bridge. Imagine you are mourning the loss of a loved one, and you find it good when you talk about your feelings. On the other hand, your partner might deal with grief by retreating inward, finding it difficult to express what they feel. Such a divergence in coping mechanisms might result in a rift between you. You might feel hurt because of their withdrawal, while they might feel overwhelmed by your requirement to talk. It is nothing less than a painful situation, but it is necessary to keep in mind that neither approach is incorrect. They are just different.

Being able to maintain open communication during this time is important. Expressing your needs to your partner while also listening to theirs can help you understand where the other is coming from. All it requires is to be patient and provide each other with the space to grieve in their own ways. By acknowledging that grief is a personal experience and that there is no one-size-fits-all method to mourn, you can foster understanding and empathy in your relationship. Take the story of Thiago and Sandra. When Thiago's father passed away, he was devastated. He found peace by keeping himself busy with work, whereas Sandra required him to talk about her feelings. At first, their different grieving styles resulted in tension and misunderstandings. Thiago felt that Sandra was pushing him to talk when he was not ready, while Sandra felt emotionally unsupported and abandoned. Understanding that their relationship was suffering, they decided to seek couple therapy. In therapy, both of them learned to communicate their requirements in the right way. Thiago expressed his requirement for time and space, and Sandra shared her need for emotional connection.

Both agreed to find a balance. Thiago would make an effort to share what he felt when he could, and Sandra would respect his need for solitude at times. With the help of this process, they found ways in which they could support one another. Thiago started to join Sandra in some of her remembrance activities, which helped him process his grief in a new way. Sandra, in turn, learned to provide Thiago with the space he required without feeling neglected. By showcasing understanding and empathy toward each other's unique grieving processes, they managed to strengthen their relationship instead of allowing grief to drive them apart. Thiago and Sandra's story highlights the importance of open communication and patience in navigating grief within a romantic relationship.

The Changing Dynamics of Friendships After Loss

The landscape of your friendships might change when you lose someone close to you. While some friends might turn out to be pillars of comfort and strength, others might find it hard to understand your grief or even keep themselves distant from you. This might turn out to be an additional layer of heartache during an already challenging time.

Friendships can turn out to be an invaluable source of support during times of grief. Some friends will step up naturally, offering you a shoulder to cry on, a listening ear, or practical help. Such friendships can make a great deal of difference, providing understanding and comfort when you require it the most. However, not all friendships might be able to withstand the strain of your grief. Some friends might not have any idea how to respond or might feel uncomfortable with the intensity of your emotions. They might try to keep themselves away from you, either emotionally or physically, which might seem like a secondary loss.

Expressing your needs in the right way during this time is important. Allow your friends to know the kind of help or support you require, whether it is help with daily tasks, someone to talk to, or simply someone to sit with you in silence. You need to be understanding in case some friends are not equipped with the kind of support you require. It is not at all a reflection of their care for you; some people simply cannot handle such heavy emotions. Research by Hogan and Greenfield sheds light on how the reactions of friends can impact those who are grieving. Their findings suggest that while some friends can provide immense support, others might end up causing more pain by being insensitive or dismissive. The research highlights the importance of seeking out those friends who can always listen without judgment and provide the kind of support that can truly help (Hogan et al., 2019). Here are some tips that can help you maintain friendships during grieving periods.

- **Open communication:** Share your needs and feelings with your friends. Always let them know how they can support you.

- **Set boundaries:** It is okay to take a step back from friends who cannot support you in the way you require.

- **Be understanding:** Understand that some friends might not have any idea how to help and might pull away. Make sure that you do not take it personally.

- **Seek supportive friends:** Try to spend time with all those friends who can provide you with understanding, empathy, and practical help.

- **Accept help:** Let your friends assist you with everyday tasks or provide company, even when it feels hard to accept help at first.

- **Forgive missteps:** Understand that friends might do or say the wrong thing at times. Try to forgive them when their intentions are good.

- **Stay connected:** Be in touch with your friends, even if it is through a phone call or a quick message.

While grief can strain even the strongest of relationships, it might also create opportunities for deeper understanding and connection. Some friends might surprise you with their depth of support and empathy, helping you develop stronger bonds that will last beyond your mourning period. True friends will be by your side through good times and bad. Trying to navigate the changing dynamics of friendships after a loss can be pretty hard. However, it is an important part of the healing process.

Interacting with Coworkers While Grieving

Trying to navigate professional relationships while grieving can turn out to be a complicated and overwhelming task. When you are dealing with the emotional fallout of a significant loss, maintaining your professional interactions and responsibilities might seem daunting. Your ability to engage, concentrate, and perform at work might be hampered. In the workplace, you might find it difficult to connect with your coworkers or focus on tasks as you did before the loss. The demands and expectations of your job might feel like a burden when you are also dealing with the weight of grief. Communicating with your employer regarding your requirements is crucial. There are workplaces that offer bereavement leave or flexible work arrangements to help you cope with this tough period.

It has been found that returning to work after a loss might trigger traumatic stress (Hurrying through Grief: Returning to Work after a Death, n.d.). In such instances, workplace support and understanding become extremely important. Your colleagues and employer play an important role in your ability to navigate grief while properly maintaining your professional life. Here are some of the challenges that you are most likely to face while managing professional relationships during a time of grief.

- **Difficulty concentrating:** Your mind is most likely to be preoccupied with the loss, making it hard to concentrate on work tasks.

- **Emotional outbursts:** You might find yourself more prone to emotional reactions, which might be a difficult thing to manage in a professional setting.

- **Decreased productivity:** The weight of grief can easily slow down your pace of work and impact your overall productivity.

- **Social withdrawal:** You might feel less inclined to engage with coworkers, resulting in isolation in the workplace.

- **Increased irritability:** Small frustrations at work might seem magnified when you are grieving, resulting in increased impatience or irritability.

Discussing your situation with supervisors or colleagues can be a sensitive but crucial step. Here's some advice on how you can approach such conversations and tips to navigate such a challenging time.

- **Be direct and honest:** When you are ready, share your situation with your supervisor and close colleagues. Let them know how grief is affecting you and what you actually need from them.

- **Set boundaries:** Try to make it clear what topics you are comfortable discussing and what is off-limits. This can help your colleagues understand how to support you without overstepping your boundaries.

- **Request flexibility:** Ask for flexible work hours or remote work options, if possible, to give yourself the time to process your grief.

- **Seek support:** Utilize any employee assistance programs (EAP) offered by your workplace. Such programs often provide counseling and other necessary resources.

- **Take breaks:** Take short breaks throughout the day to manage your emotions and cut down on stress.

- **Keep communication open:** Update your senior on a daily basis regarding your progress and any adjustments that you might require to your tasks or work schedule.

- **Practice self-care:** Make sure that you take proper care of your mental and physical health outside of work. This can help take care of the emotional toll of grief.

- **Lean on trusted colleagues:** Identify colleagues who can provide support and understanding. Having someone to talk to can make a huge difference.

- **Plan for trigger days:** Be aware of events or dates that might be particularly challenging and make plans accordingly. You can communicate this with your senior if required.

By being honest and open about your challenges and needs, you can create a supportive work environment that acknowledges your grief while letting you maintain your professional responsibilities.

Dealing with Insensitive Reactions from Others

Navigating grief is hard enough without the extra challenge of dealing with insensitive reactions from other people. Unfortunately, it is common for people who are well-meaning to unintentionally use misguided comments that might feel dismissive or minimizing. Some might tell you to "stay strong" or "move on" too soon, while others might try to downplay your loss by comparing it to less significant experiences. Such reactions can turn out to be hurtful and can make an already difficult time even harder to bear. During my journey through grief, I found it important to set clear boundaries so that I could protect my emotional well-being. It is okay to limit your interactions with all those who cannot offer the kind of support you require. Trying to prioritize your mental health is not selfish. It is a crucial step in healing. Make the effort to surround yourself with people who truly understand and support you. Do not think twice about stepping back from those who don't. Let's have a look at some strategies to deal with insensitive reactions.

- **Communicate what you need:** If someone's behavior or comment is hurtful, let them know in a gentle way. You can say something like, "I appreciate your concern, but what I truly need now is someone who can just listen to me," or "It is important for me to take my time with this process."

- **Set boundaries:** It is okay to limit your time with or distance yourself from all those who keep making you feel worse. You can say, "I am not ready to talk about such things right now," or "I need some space to process what I feel."

- **Seek understanding allies:** Try to keep yourself surrounded by people who can truly understand what you are going through. This could be family, friends, or support groups where you can share what you feel without any fear of dismissal or judgment.

- **Have a supportive script ready:** You can prepare a few responses for when you come across insensitive comments. Phrases such as "Everyone grieves differently, and this is what I need at the moment," can help deflect unwelcome advice without causing confrontation.

- **Practice self-care:** Make sure that you take time for activities that nurture your soul and help you feel grounded. This could include spending some time in nature, reading, or engaging in creative hobbies.

- **Know it is okay to say "no":** There is no need to accept every invitation or participate in all kinds of conversation. Protecting your emotional health, at times, means saying no to all those things that feel excessively overwhelming.

The "Empathy Shortcut" for Connecting Despite Grief

Trying to navigate through the waves of grief, I discovered what I like to call the "empathy shortcut". It is a method that can help you connect with others easily, even amidst the chaos of grief. This shortcut is rooted in the profound understanding and shared experience that come from facing the same kinds of losses. When grief leaves you feeling isolated, finding common ground with other people who have sustained similar pain can turn out to be extremely comforting. Empathy comes with a unique power to fill gaps in communication and understanding. When we showcase empathy, we are essentially saying, "I can see your pain, and I am right here with you." This kind of profound acknowledgement can help in the creation of a deep sense of validation and connection. In my own experience, meeting other people who had lost their loved ones helped me understand that I was not alone. Even if these individuals were strangers, the shared grief experience developed an instant bond.

Despite all kinds of challenges that grief brings to your relationships, it can also develop opportunities for better understanding and connection. The empathy shortcut refers to all those ways in which shared experiences of loss can help foster a sense of immediate connection. When you come across someone who has also walked a similar path of loss, you might find that you can relate to one another on a profound level. It is more like an unspoken language, a mutual understanding that does not need justifications or lengthy explanations. For instance, I remember attending a support group where I met someone who had also lost someone close in their life. Despite having never met before, our shared experiences of loss made it easy to connect. There was no need to explain the depth of our pain. It was understood. Such a connection provided immense comfort and support as I also tried to navigate my grief journey.

These connections can turn out to be a source of solace, providing comfort that you are not alone in your struggles. They serve to provide a unique kind of support that even family members and close friends might not be able to deliver. This is the essence of the empathy shortcut. As you keep walking on your path through grief, keep in mind that while it can impact your current relationships, it can also offer the potential for new and meaningful connections.

Chapter 5:
Grief and Your Identity

Grief does not change you. It reveals you.
–John Green

When you lose someone close to you, it does not only break your heart - it might also shake the very core of who you are. This section explores how grief can impact your sense of identity. As you lose a loved one, the person you were when you were with them and the kind of life you shared together might feel like it's been torn away. This can leave you questioning who you are and how you can move forward in life. I remember talking to Anton, a man who lost his wife of 40 years. Anton was not only mourning the loss of his partner but also dealing with his own sense of self. They had always been "Anton and Angel", a duo whose lives were deeply intertwined. After Angel's death, he found himself lost, unsure of who he was without her. The activities they enjoyed together, the routines they shared, and even his own preferences and habits seemed to have no meaning. It was as if a part of his identity had vanished along with her. This section delves into stories like Anton's, examining how grief can change our identities.

Grief's Assault on Your Sense of Self

Grief can easily disrupt your sense of self, leaving you feeling unfamiliar even to yourself. When you lose someone close to you, it is not only their absence that you mourn but also the part of your identity that was intertwined with theirs. Such a disruption might manifest in several ways, often making you feel like a completely different person or making it hard to recognize yourself. I have seen this in various conversations with those who have lost their loved ones. One man, Denver, spoke about how he felt like a shadow of his former self when his wife passed away. They had shared so much of their lives together that, without her, he felt incomplete and lost. Daily activities and routines that once brought joy now seem purposeless. Such a shift in identity is common and might turn out to be deeply unsettling.

Different people tend to experience such disruptions in unique ways. Some might feel a sense of alienation from their own lives, as if they are doing nothing other than watching themselves from the outside. Others might feel that they have lost touch with their core beliefs and values, questioning who they are in the absence of their loved ones. For some, this disorientation might result in feelings like they are living the life of someone else, not being able to connect with their previous sense of self. The psychological impact of spousal loss has been studied deeply. According to research, the death of a spouse might trigger significant depressive symptoms and impact one's mental health. This study also highlights how our sense of self can be intertwined with our partners and how their loss can result in a profound identity crisis (Utz et al., 2011).

Trying to navigate this identity disruption might require immense self-compassion and patience. It is necessary to acknowledge that it is completely normal to feel lost and to give yourself permission to grieve not just the person who has died but also the version of yourself that existed with them. Seeking support from family, friends, or a therapist can be crucial during this time. They can provide you with the necessary help to process your feelings and start to explore who you are now in the absence of your loved one. Keep in mind that rediscovering your sense of self is a gradual process. It involves developing new routines, connections, and interests that can resonate with the present reality. While you might not be able to feel exactly like your old self again, this journey can lead to a new understanding of the person you are.

Masculinity and the Pressure to "Be Strong"

Navigating grief as a man often comes with an extra layer of complexity because of societal expectations. There exists this pervasive notion that men are required to "be strong," suppressing what they feel to maintain a facade of resilience. Such expectations can complicate the grieving process for men to a great extent. I have seen how this pressure to conform to traditional masculinity can hamper genuine emotional expression. When I lost my father, I felt an overwhelming urge to appear strong, not only for myself but for those around me. Crying seemed like a betrayal of my role as the strong pillar of the family. However, beneath the exterior, I was struggling considerably, feeling isolated by my inability to mourn openly. Society often sees emotional expression in men as a sign of weakness. From a very young age, boys are conditioned to believe that showcasing vulnerability is not at all acceptable. Phrases such as "boys don't cry" or "man up" are drilled into our subconscious, giving shape to the way in which we deal with emotions later in life. When we get hit by grief, this ingrained behavior can make it hard to process loss in a healthy way.

There's a study that delves into such traditional ideologies of masculinity. This research illustrates how men are often trapped by societal norms that dictate they must remain stoic, even when faced with profound loss. Such suppression of emotions does not only complicate grief but can also lead to serious psychological problems like anxiety and depression (Pederson & Vogel, 2007). One of my friends, Mike, struggled a lot after losing his sister. He felt the weight of expectation to stay strong for his family, never letting himself have the space to grieve openly. With time, this unaddressed grief started to manifest as frustration and anger, straining all his relationships. Furthermore, it impacted his mental health. It was not until he sought therapy did he start to understand the importance of expressing his emotions.

In order to navigate such challenges, it is important that you start redefining what it means to be strong. Strength does not lie in suppressing emotions but in having the capacity and courage to confront them head-on. Acknowledging what you feel, whether by talking to a trusted friend, joining a support group, or seeking professional help, can be regarded as a sign of true resilience. Developing a space where it is acceptable to express grief can also break down such damaging stereotypes. Encouraging open conversations about emotions, especially among men, can pave the way for a healthier grieving process. It is about giving yourself the grace - to feel, mourn, and heal without any extra weight of societal expectations.

Finding Yourself Again After Loss

Experiencing loss can leave you feeling like a part of yourself is missing, and the journey to rediscover yourself can be daunting. I have been through it myself, and I know very well how disorienting it can feel. However, there are steps that you can take to find your way back to a sense of self, even after experiencing a profound loss. Here are some strategies that can help:

- **Journaling:** Writing down your feelings and thoughts can turn out to be extremely therapeutic. It is a way to process your emotions, reflect on the journey, and start to understand how the loss might have impacted you. Journaling can serve as a personal conversation with yourself, helping you make sense of your new reality.

- **Counseling and therapy:** Speaking with a professional can provide you with a safe space to explore your feelings. Counselors and therapists are trained to help you navigate the complexity of loss and grief. They can provide coping strategies and help you work through all kinds of emotions that arise.

- **Support groups:** Joining a group of people who are going through similar experiences can be comforting. Hearing the stories of other people and sharing your own can help create a sense of understanding and community. Support groups can remind you that you are not alone in your grief.

- **Self-care:** Focus on activities that can nurture your soul and body. This can include meditation, exercise, engaging in hobbies you love, or spending time in nature. Taking care of your physical health can impact your emotional well-being in a positive way.

- **Meditation and mindfulness:** Practicing mindfulness can help you stay present and can cut down on anxiety. Meditation can provide you with a sense of calm and help you connect with your inner self. Such practices can provide an escape from the turmoil of grief.

- **Connecting with loved ones:** Spend time with friends and family members who support you. Sharing memories of your loved one and talking about your feelings can be healing. Let other people be there for you, and do not be afraid to ask for help when you require it.

- **Develop new routines:** Establishing new routines can bring a sense of stability and normalcy. This does not indicate forgetting your loved one. It is all about finding a new rhythm that incorporates your memories while letting you move ahead in life.

- **Exploring creative outlets:** Take part in activities that will let you express your emotions in a creative way. Whether it is music, painting, writing, or other forms of art, creative expression can be a superb way to process grief.

- **Setting small goals:** Try to take things one step at a time. Do not rush with your goals. Celebrate the small wins as you navigate your path to healing.

Rediscovering yourself after a huge loss is a personal journey. It will take patience, time, and self-compassion. Be gentle with yourself as you try to navigate this new terrain.

Post-Traumatic Growth: How Grief Can Change You for the Better

There is no doubt that grief is an overwhelming force that can disrupt every aspect of one's life. However, amidst the pain and sorrow, there lies the potential for something truly transformative: post-traumatic growth. This concept refers to the positive changes that can emerge from a struggle with a major life crisis or traumatic event. Post-traumatic growth does not indicate that the grief will disappear or that the loss will become any less significant. Rather, it signifies that through enduring such hardship, you might get to find new perspectives, strengths, and a deeper appreciation for life. It is about finding a way to grow and rebuild in the aftermath of a tragedy.

Take the example of a man named Travis, who lost his wife unexpectedly. Initially, Travis was engulfed in a sea of despair, feeling that his world had come to a cruel and abrupt end. The grief was unbearable, and for a long period of time, he was not able to see a way ahead. However, as time passed, he started to notice subtle shifts in himself. Travis found a new sense of purpose in volunteering at a local hospice, where he provided comfort to others facing similar losses. Such an experience not only helped him process his grief but also ignited a passion for helping other people; a passion he had never realized before. Through this journey, Travis experienced what psychologists refer to as post-traumatic growth. He developed a greater appreciation for life, a stronger sense of personal strength, and a newfound ability to connect deeply with other people. The loss of his wife remained a painful chapter in his life, but it also turned out to be a catalyst for positive transformation.

Another such example is Mike, who lost his best friend in a tragic accident. Mike was completely devastated, and the grief was compounded by a sense of helplessness and guilt. However, with the help of therapy and support groups, Mike started to channel his pain into advocacy. He started a foundation in the name of his friend to raise awareness about road safety. This endeavor not only honored the memory of his friend but also provided Mike with a sense of purpose and a way to make some difference in the world. Such stories illustrate that, while grief can be quite painful, it also has the potential to lead to significant personal growth. It has been found that people who experience post-traumatic growth often report improved personal strength, better relationships, a deeper sense of spirituality, and a greater appreciation for life (Zoellner & Maercker, 2006). If you are dealing with grief, it might feel impossible to imagine any sort of positive outcome. That is okay. Post-traumatic growth won't happen overnight, and it is not a linear process. It is about finding purpose and meaning in the face of loss, even when it takes time. You can consider the following steps to nurture this growth:

- **Engage in meaningful activities:** Find ways in which you can honor the memory of your loved one or contribute to a cause that resonates with you.

- **Seek support:** Keep yourself surrounded by people who support your journey. Support groups can be helpful.

- **Reflect on your journey:** Let yourself take the time to reflect on how the experience has changed you. Talking with a therapist or journaling can help.

- **Embrace new perspectives:** Be open to new ways of living and thinking that might emerge from your experience.

It is possible to rebuild your identity after experiencing a loss in life. Just be patient with yourself.

Chapter 6:
Healthy Coping Strategies

When someone you love becomes a memory, the memory becomes a treasure.
–Unknown

Dealing with grief is never easy, especially as a man in a society that always expects you to be strong by suppressing your emotions. I understand how overwhelming and isolating this might feel. This chapter is dedicated to exploring healthy coping strategies that can help you navigate through this hard time. Understanding the importance of these strategies is crucial. They are not about forgetting or moving on, but about finding ways to live with your loss and keep moving ahead in life.

The Importance of Accepting Your Feelings and Constructive Ways to Release Anger and Frustration

Losing someone close to you can trigger a wide range of emotions. You might feel anger, sadness, guilt, or even confusion. It is important to acknowledge and accept such feelings instead of pushing them away. When you deny your feelings, you are not only avoiding the pain. You will also be avoiding the process of healing. Grief is not an issue to be solved but a journey to be experienced. Embracing your emotions will let you move through your grief more naturally. It will let you honor your loss and start the slow process of finding a new normal. It is completely okay to feel overwhelmed. It is okay to feel lost, to be angry, or to cry. By accepting these emotions, you will give yourself permission to grieve in your own way, without judgment.

When you grieve, it is common to feel frustration and anger bubbling to the surface. Such emotions can catch you off guard and leave you wondering why you are feeling this way. Anger is a natural response to loss, often stemming from a sense of injustice, helplessness, or guilt. Recognizing this can be the first step in the management of the same in a constructive way. During my journey through grief, I found that channeling my anger into creative outlets and physical activities made a huge difference. Let's have a look at some strategies that can help you release those intense emotions in a healthy way:

- **Exercise:** Engaging in physical activities such as boxing, running, or weightlifting, can provide a powerful outlet for your anger. The physical exertion can help burn off some of the pent-up energy and can make you feel calmer and more centered.

- **Artistic expression:** Creating something can turn out to be extremely therapeutic. Whether it is drawing, painting, or sculpting, expressing your feelings through art will let you process your emotions in a non-verbal way.

- **Writing:** Writing letters to your loved ones, drafting unsent letters, or simply documenting your experiences and thoughts can help clarify your emotions and provide a sense of release from what is bottled up inside.

- **Music:** Singing, playing an instrument, or even simply listening to music that resonates with your feelings can be an intuitive way to process and release anger. Music has a unique way of touching our emotions and helping us to express what we might not be able to put into words.

- **Gardening:** Connecting with nature with the help of gardening can be very effective. The physical activity involved in digging, planting, and tending to plants can be a peaceful way to channel your emotions.

- **DIY projects:** Engaging in hands-on projects such as home improvement, woodworking, or crafting can provide a constructive outlet for your frustration. The effort and focus required for such activities can also provide a distraction from your grief.

How to Let Yourself Cry

Crying is often seen as a sign of weakness, especially when it comes to men. However, it is a natural and healthy response to pain. It is a physical manifestation of the deep emotional turmoil you are experiencing. Letting yourself cry can be relieving, providing a necessary release for the overwhelming emotions that generally come with grief. I have been there, feeling the pressure to hold back tears, thinking it will make me stronger. The truth is that crying is a form of strength. It takes courage to be vulnerable and to let your true feelings surface. Holding everything in will only prolong the pain and result in more serious emotional problems down the line. There are studies that show the therapeutic effects of crying. It has been found that crying can help lower blood pressure, reduce stress, and release toxins from the body. When you cry, your body releases endorphins, which act like natural painkillers, and oxytocin, which can help enhance mood and promote a sense of calm (Gross et al., 1994).

Do let yourself cry when you feel the need. Find a safe space where you can be comfortable letting your emotions out. This might be in the privacy of your home, during a quiet walk in nature, or even in the shower, where the sound of water can be soothing. Keep in mind that crying is not a sign of defeat. It is a natural process that can help you heal. It is alright to show your emotions and grieve openly. You are not required to hide your pain or pretend to be okay when you are not. By embracing your tears, you can acknowledge your grief and let yourself process it in a healthy way.

The Healing Importance of Remembrance and Ritual

Finding ways to honor and remember your loved one can be a profound part of the healing process. Remembrance and rituals can provide a sense of connection and continuity, letting you hold onto the memory of the person you have lost while moving ahead in your own life. The healing importance of remembrance and ritual cannot be overstated. It is said that rituals can offer a structured way to express grief, find comfort, and share memories (The Role of Rituals in the Grieving Process, n.d.). Such rituals can take various forms, from traditional ceremonies to personal practices that hold special meaning for you. I have found that creating and participating in rituals helped me process my grief. Whether it is visiting a significant place, lighting a candle, or simply taking a moment every day to reflect, such acts can bring a sense of solace and peace. They serve as a tangible way to honor the legacy of your loved one and keep their memory alive.

Rituals can also provide a sense of control at a time when everything else feels chaotic. They provide a way to channel your emotions and find moments of calm amidst the storm. Additionally, engaging in rituals with friends and family can help improve bonds and develop a shared space for collective support and mourning. It is necessary to keep in mind that there is no correct or incorrect way to commemorate your loved one. The rituals you opt for need to resonate with you personally and reflect the unique relationship you had. There are people who find comfort in traditional religious or cultural ceremonies, while others might prefer more creative and personal expressions of remembrance. Embracing rituals as a part of the grieving process can help navigate the complicated emotions that come with loss. They will let you celebrate the life of your loved one and find meaning in their absence. By integrating such practices into your life, you can create a bridge between the past and the future, honoring the memories and love that will be a part of you all the time.

Grief Journaling for Clarity and Catharsis

Grief journaling can be a powerful tool for gaining clarity and achieving catharsis during difficult times. When I first started journaling after my loss, I found it to be a safe space where I could pour out all my thoughts and emotions without any kind of judgment. It helped me process my grief in a way that conversations with other people sometimes couldn't. In order to get started with grief journaling, there is no need for any kind of fancy equipment. All you need is a notebook and a pen. Start by setting aside a few minutes every day, preferably at a time when you know you will not be interrupted. Write about everything that comes to your mind. It could be memories of your loved one, the challenges you are facing, or the emotions you are experiencing. The key here is to be honest and allow your thoughts to flow freely.

Incorporating such a practice into your daily life can be easy. I found it helpful to make journaling part of my morning or evening routine. If you are not sure what to write about, try prompts such as "Today, I miss you because..." or "I remember when we...". This can help you get started and keep the process from feeling overwhelming. Grief journaling is not about producing perfect prose. It is about providing yourself with a reflective and private space to process what you feel and find some relief.

Making Self-Care a Priority

Making self-care a priority might feel challenging, especially when you are in the depths of grief. I remember struggling with the idea that it was okay to take time for myself when everything felt so heavy. However, I have learned that self-care is not a luxury. It is a necessary component of healing. Incorporating self-care into your everyday life can start with small and manageable steps. For me, it started with setting aside just a few minutes every day to do something that nurtured my well-being. This could be as simple as taking a walk in the park, listening to a favorite piece of music, or enjoying a quiet cup of tea.

It could be helpful to establish a routine that includes self-care activities. Schedule time for things that bring you relaxation and peace. Whether it is taking a warm bath, reading a book, or practicing a hobby you love, such moments can provide you with a much-needed break from the intensity of grief. Keep in mind that self-care is about listening to your mind and body, and responding with kindness. Provide yourself permission to rest when you feel tired, eat healthy food, and seek support from professionals or friends if required. Prioritizing self-care can help rebuild your resilience and strength, letting you navigate the journey of grief a bit more easily.

Nutrition and Exercise Helps With Grief

When you deal with grief, taking care of your body might feel like an afterthought. However, I have found that focusing on nutrition and exercise can make a huge difference in how you deal with weight loss. Nourishing your body in the right way and staying active can help stabilize your mood and provide a sense of routine during such a tough time. In terms of nutrition, concentrate on balanced meals that include various kinds of veggies, fruits, whole grains, and lean meats. It is easy to fall into the trap of comfort eating or skipping meals. However, maintaining a healthy diet can help maintain steady energy levels. Simple changes such as drinking plenty of water, eating smaller, more frequent meals, and reducing sugar intake can support your emotional and physical health.

Exercise, even in small amounts, can turn out to be helpful. It does not have to be anything intense. Some gentle stretching, a short walk, or even a few minutes of yoga can help. Physical activity can help release endorphins, which can improve your mood and help you deal with the sadness and fatigue often associated with grief. Incorporating such habits into your daily life might seem like a huge thing, but starting small can help. Prepare nutritious and simple meals and set aside time every day for some form of movement, no matter how light it is.

Sleep Strategies and Routines as Anchors

I know firsthand how grief can rob you of sleep, leaving you overwhelmed and exhausted. During such sleepless nights, it feels like your mind won't stop racing, replaying worries and memories. This lack of rest only makes it difficult to face the day and manage your emotions. However, there are strategies that can help, providing a sense of stability and some relief. First, try to create a bedtime routine that can signal your body and mind that it is time to wind down. This can be as simple as turning off electronics an hour before going to bed, dimming the lights, and engaging in calming activities such as listening to soft music or reading. Stay away from stimulants, such as caffeine, and heavy meals in the evening. It can help prepare your body for rest.

Another crucial step is establishing a consistent sleep schedule. Going to bed and getting up at the same time on a daily basis, even on weekends, can help regulate your internal clock. It might take some time to adjust, but persistence is key. With time, this routine can turn out to be a comforting anchor, providing a significant sense of predictability amidst all the chaos of grief. Incorporating relaxation techniques before going to bed can make a huge difference. Progressive muscle relaxation, deep breathing exercises, or guided imagery can help calm your mind and reduce physical tension. There are various online resources and apps that provide guided sessions to help you get started.

Another practical tip is to create a sleep-friendly environment. Make your bedroom a sanctuary dedicated to rest. Keep the room dark, cool, and quiet. Investing in a comfortable mattress and pillows can help. If outside noise is a problem, you can consider using earplugs. It is necessary to be gentle with yourself during this time. If you find that you cannot sleep, do not stress much about it. At times, getting out of bed and engaging in a non-stimulating and quiet activity can help rest your mind. Get back to bed only when you feel sleepy again. Routines extend beyond bedtime as well. Daily rituals can provide a sense of normalcy and structure. Whether it is a cup of tea in the early afternoon, a morning walk, or a phone call with a friend, such small routines can serve as comforting anchors. They can provide a sense of stability and control when everything else in life feels uncertain.

Staying Connected to Avoid Isolation and Discovering New Purpose

Grief can often result in a profound sense of isolation, making it hard to reach out and staying connected with other people. Yet, maintaining social connections is important during this hard time. It is easy to retreat into yourself, but isolation can amplify feelings of loneliness and make the process of healing even harder. I remember speaking with Brett, whose daughter had a deadly disease. He shared how isolating it felt despite having family and friends around. He said, "I wanted to shut everyone out. However, the more I did, the more I felt trapped in my own sorrow." Brett's experience is not uncommon. It is a natural response to want to withdraw, but it is equally important to fight against this impulse.

Staying connected does not mean that you will need to be constantly social or put on a brave face. It can be as simple as being in touch with close friends or even participating in online forums where you can share your feelings with other people who understand. If reaching out feels daunting, start small. Send a text message to a friend or family member, letting them know you are thinking of them. Schedule a daily phone call or a coffee chat. Being proactive in maintaining such connections can provide a sense of support and normalcy. Even when it is hard to open up, the act of being around other people can be comforting.

Engaging in community activities can also help. Joining a club or group with similar interests or volunteering can offer a sense of belonging and purpose. It might feel quite challenging to think about giving back when you are grieving, but many find that helping others provides a sense of fulfillment and a new perspective. For instance, Brett started volunteering at a local NGO. He found that helping others through their own hard times gave him a sense of connection and purpose. Rediscovering a sense of purpose is another important aspect of staying connected. After a significant loss, it is common to feel adrift and uncertain about the future. Taking up a project, exploring new hobbies, or setting small goals can be useful.

Most importantly, asking for help is necessary when you truly need it. There is often a stigma, particularly for men, around seeking support. Society tends to value self-reliance, making it feel like asking for help is a sign of weakness. It is important to understand that asking for help is not only okay but also necessary. Grief can be a heavy burden to carry alone. Reaching out is a crucial step in the healing process. People around you often want to help but might not know how. By expressing your requirements, you give them the chance to support you in meaningful ways. While grief might feel overwhelming, employing the strategies that we discussed in this section can make things more manageable.

Chapter 7:
The Importance of Processing Your Loss

When you are sorrowful look again in your heart, and you shall see that in truth you are weeping for that which has been your delight.
–Kahlil Gibran

Grief is an overwhelming experience, and being able to process your loss is an important step in healing. In this section, we will explore what it means to truly process a loss and why it is so crucial in the grieving journey. Processing a loss involves confronting your emotions, understanding your pain, and finding useful ways in which you can move ahead in life without forgetting the love you shared. Suppressing or ignoring your feelings might seem like the best way to cope, but it will lead to more pain down the line. When you let yourself fully experience and process your grief, you can open the door to true healing. This chapter aims to guide you through this hard process, offering strategies and insights to help you navigate the stormy seas of grief. Processing your loss is not about "getting over" it but about finding a way to live with it and eventually find peace amidst all the sorrow.

Telling the Story of Your Loved One and the Importance of Facing Pain

Grief is a journey that everyone takes in their own way. One of the most powerful methods of processing grief is storytelling. Sharing stories about your loved one can turn out to be extremely therapeutic, as it will let you keep their memory alive and honor their impact on your own life. It has been found that narrating the story of a loved one's life and death can help make sense of the loss and integrate it into your life story (Neimeyer, 2005). When my friend Jerome lost his mother, he found solace in sharing her stories. He would recount her vibrant personality, her profound love for gardening, and the tiny, everyday moments they shared. Such stories became a way for Jerome to feel connected to his mother and to process his grief. It was not only about remembering her; it was about finding a way to live with her absence while still celebrating her presence in his life. Talking about your loved one can help externalize the grief, making things more manageable. It transforms a solitary, internal pain into a shared experience. It can create a space for understanding and support. This process can help you organize your feelings and thoughts, making the chaos of grief a bit more structured.

However, it is a natural thing to want to avoid pain. We think that this will help us cope. What we fail to understand is that avoiding the pain only prolongs the process of grieving. The Dual Process Model of Coping with Bereavement by Stroebe and Schut focuses on the importance of oscillating between confronting the loss and taking breaks from extreme emotions (Stroebe & Schut, 1999). Facing the pain will let you process it, while avoidance can lead to unresolved grief and emotional distress. Avoidance might seem like the best way to protect yourself, but it often results in more profound and lasting pain. I recall a story from a man named Jake who lost his sister suddenly. For years, Jake threw himself into work, avoiding all kinds of reminders or thoughts of his sister. Eventually, the unaddressed grief caught up with him, manifesting in depression and anxiety. It wasn't until Jake started to face his pain by talking about his sister, visiting the places they loved, and letting himself cry that he started to heal.

Facing your pain is not at all about forcing yourself to be sad. It is about letting yourself feel whatever comes up and recognizing that such feelings are a natural part of the grieving process. It is about striking the right balance between honoring the memory of your loved one and taking care of your emotional well-being. You can transform your sorrow into a testament of resilience and love, making sure that the legacy of your loved one continues to shine through your life.

Continuing Bonds: Redefining Your Relationship

Maintaining a bond with a deceased loved one can be an important part of the healing process. It is said that keeping a connection with the person who has passed can provide comfort and help integrate the loss into your life in a healthy way (Klass, 2006). After Joseph's father passed away, he found himself talking to him during quiet moments, especially when he faced challenges or required guidance. It felt like he was still with him, offering his support and wisdom. This ongoing connection did not stop him from grieving. In fact, it gave him a sense of comfort and continuity.

There are various ways in which this bond can be maintained. Keeping photos of your loved ones around your home can be a simple and powerful reminder of their presence in your life. Such images can evoke stories and memories, keeping their spirit alive in your everyday routine. Celebrating their lives on special occasions can be meaningful. Whether it is their anniversary, birthday, or a significant holiday, taking time to honor their memory can provide a sense of closeness. For instance, I light a candle for my father every year on his birthday, sharing stories and reflecting on our time together. It is a kind of ritual that brings both joy and a bittersweet reminder of his absence. Creating personal traditions can help as well. Some people find solace in visiting the favorite spot of their loved one, cooking their favorite meal, or listening to their favorite music. Such actions are small yet powerful ways to keep their essence a part of your life.

Continuing bonds are all about redefining your relationship with the deceased, not letting go of it. It is more like an acknowledgment that love and connection do not end with death.

Coping With Birthdays, Holidays and Anniversaries

Birthdays, holidays, and anniversaries can be some of the hardest days when you are grieving. Such times are traditionally filled with togetherness and joy, but in the absence of your loved one, they can turn out to be painful reminders of your loss. A practical approach to dealing with this is to plan ahead. Anticipate these days and think about how you might want to spend them. It is completely okay to acknowledge that such days will be difficult. Give yourself permission to feel all kinds of emotions that come up, and do not feel pressured to conform to any expectations.

Some men might find solace in creating new traditions. I remember talking to Tom, who lost his wife a few years ago. On her birthday, in place of their usual celebration, he decided to spend the day doing all those activities she loved. He went hiking in her favorite spot and also cooked her favorite meal for dinner. This ritual not only helped Tom honor her memory but also provided him with a sense of purpose and connection on an otherwise hard day. Another great way to cope is to involve other people. Sharing memories and stories with friends or family can provide comfort. Thiago, who lost his best friend, found that organizing a small gathering of close friends every year on his best friend's birthday helped him. They would share stories, cry, laugh, and share his best friend's life. This kind of communal remembrance provided a support system and a way to celebrate the legacy of Thiago's best friend.

Some men might prefer a quieter approach. Samuel, who lost both his parents in a pandemic, chooses to spend these days in reflection. He visits the graves of his parents, brings flowers, and spends some time alone in silence, talking to his mother and father in his heart and mind. This private ritual helps him process his grief and feel a constant bond with his parents. Whatever method feels right for you, the key is to strike the right balance that honors your loved one while also taking proper care of your emotional requirements. Listen to yourself, be kind to yourself, and do what feels most true to your heart.

Dealing With Your Loved One's Belongings

Sorting through the belongings of a loved one, can be one of the most emotionally challenging aspects of grieving. Every item holds a story or a memory, and deciding what to do with such possessions can feel overwhelming. I remember when a close friend of mine, Samuel, lost his wife. He shared how paralyzing it felt when he walked into their shared closet, saw her clothes, and felt the weight of her absence. This deep attachment to the physical reminders of our loved ones is a common experience. One strategy that might help is to take your time. There is no need to rush through everything at once. Start with small steps, maybe a single box or a drawer. Let yourself feel the emotions that come with every item, and understand that this is a natural part of grief.

Some people tend to find comfort in donating items. Samuel eventually decided to donate the clothes of his wife to a local shelter. It gave him solace to know that her belongings would help other people in need. In case donation feels too hard for you, you can think of repurposing items. A shirt could become a quilt, or jewelry could be turned into a new piece. Preserving items as keepsakes can be another meaningful approach. Creating a memory box with special items or framing favorite photographs can provide a tangible connection to your loved one. When I went through my father's things, I kept his watch and a few of his books. These items now have a special place in my home, serving as a comforting reminder of him.

Your loved one's online social media accounts will also require decision-making if these should continue to exist or not. Once again, it is best to take your time as these may hold a treasure-trove of memories and once removed are usually irretrievable.

The key here is to determine the method that feels right for you. There is no right way to handle this process. Have faith in your instincts, take it one step at a time, and be gentle with yourself as you try to navigate this personal journey.

Visiting Special Places of Remembrance

Visiting places that hold special significance to your loved one can be a healing way to process grief. Such locations can serve as physical anchors to your memories, helping you feel closer to your loved one. When my friend Mike lost his son, he often visited the park where they used to play together. He found that being in that familiar setting brought back vivid memories of their laughter and conversations. Sitting on their favorite bench, he felt a sense of connection and peace, as if he were still with him in some way. Such visits can also provide a space for reflection and quiet contemplation. After my father passed away, I started visiting his favorite fishing spot by the lake. It became a sanctuary for me, a place where I could fondly remember him and process my emotions away from the distractions of everyday life. Each visit felt like a small step in the direction of healing, a way to keep his memory alive while finding comfort in his routine.

You can consider setting aside specific days to visit such meaningful places. Whether it is a favorite café, a special beach, or a frequented hiking trail, such spots can become touchstones in your journey through grief. They remind you of the experiences and love you shared, providing a tangible connection to your loved one's presence. Each visit is an opportunity to honor their memory and to give yourself permission to feel whatever comes up. Grief is a process, and such moments of remembrance can be healing opportunities.

The "Grief Release" Method for Letting Go

The 'grief release' method can turn out to be a powerful tool when it comes to processing grief and finding peace. This approach involves acknowledging and expressing your feelings, which can help get rid of the intense pain associated with loss. The first step is to develop a safe space where you can feel comfortable expressing your emotions. This could be a quiet room in your house, during a therapy session, or a peaceful outdoor spot. It is important to feel secure and free from judgment in this space. Let yourself fully experience your grief. This might involve writing a letter to your loved one, speaking out loud to them as if they are present in front of you, or simply allowing your emotions to flow freely. In his book "Grief Counseling and Grief Therapy," J. William Worden emphasizes the importance of actively mourning. By giving voice to your anger, sorrow, or confusion, you can start processing such emotions instead of keeping them bottled up.

Another important step is to reflect on your memories and the significance of your loved one's life. Look at photos, share stories, or create a memory book. This will not only help honor their memory, but it can also help you process your feelings and start to find meaning in the loss. By letting yourself fully experience and express your grief, you can start healing and carry the memory of your loved one forward with resilience and love.

Finding Peace and Acceptance

Finding peace and acceptance after losing a loved one is a profound journey. It is necessary to understand that acceptance does not mean forgetting or moving on as if nothing happened. Instead, it means learning to live with the loss and integrating it into your life in a way that honors your loved one's memory while letting you heal. Acceptance means acknowledging the reality of the loss and understanding that your life has changed. It can be said that those who reach acceptance often feel a sense of peace. They can cherish the good memories without getting overwhelmed by the pain. This does not indicate that the grief disappears, but it becomes a part of your story. Remember the happy times, talk about your feelings, and slowly let yourself engage with life again. It is a gradual process, and it is okay to take your time. You will have to find a new way to live and keep the memory of your loved one alive while embracing the present.

When it comes to grief, it is natural to feel stuck at times. How can someone get rid of this stuck feeling and move ahead in life with the memories of their loved one? I will show you how to do so in the next section.

Chapter 8: Feeling Stuck

We must embrace pain and burn it as fuel for our journey.
–Kenji Miyazawa

Feeling stuck in grief is something many of us experience, and it is more common than you might think. Grief might seem like an endless loop, where the sadness and pain seem insurmountable, trapping you in a cycle of heartache. I remember talking to my friend Dave after he lost his brother. For months, he could not move past the overwhelming sense of loss. Every day felt like a struggle, and he often said that he felt like he was sinking into quicksand. Dave could not understand why he could not move ahead in life and why the pain was not lessening with time. His story is a testament to the reality that grief is not a linear process. Feeling stuck does not indicate that you are failing or that something is wrong with you. It is a part of the journey.

Myths and Misconceptions About Grief

Many of us have encountered myths and misconceptions about grief that can make the grieving journey even harder. You have probably come across things like "grief has a timeline" or "men don't cry." Such ideas might lead to unrealistic expectations and add to the pressure you are already feeling. Many believe that you should be "over it" after a few months, but the truth is that grief is a deeply personal process with no fixed endpoint. Everyone grieves differently at their own pace. There's a common misconception that you should move on quickly and not dwell on the past. This can pressure people to hide their feelings and pretend that they are completely okay, which is not healthy at all. It is necessary to keep in mind that grieving is a natural response to loss, and it is okay when you take your time.

There is another belief that being strong means not showcasing your emotions. Society often expects men to be stoic, but suppressing emotions can result in significant issues down the line. Some people think that avoiding reminders of their loved ones can help them forget the pain. However, this kind of avoidance might end up prolonging the grieving process. Facing the pain and remembering the loved one can be important steps in the direction of healing. Lastly, people often assume that once you have reached acceptance, the grief is over. Acceptance does not indicate the end of grief. It means integrating the loss into your life. You can still have moments of longing and sadness, and that is okay. Understanding such myths can help you navigate grief in a compassionate way. It is important to let yourself grieve in your own way and get help when needed.

What to Do When Grief Feels Unbearable

Grief can sometimes feel like a crushing weight, making it harder for you to breathe freely or find the will to keep going in life. When grief turns out to be unbearable, it is important that you find ways in which you can cope and help you through the darkest moments. One of the most crucial things you can do is reach out for support. Talk to a family member, a trusted friend, or a grief counselor who can provide you with a listening ear and understanding. Let yourself cry and express what you feel. Bottling up your feelings might end up intensifying the pain. Allowing yourself to grieve openly can help. It is okay to feel vulnerable and to let others see your pain.

Developing a routine can provide you with a sense of stability. Even simple tasks like making your bed or cooking a meal can offer you a sense of normalcy and control in the midst of all the chaos. Engaging in activities that connect you with your loved one can be comforting. Writing letters to them, looking through their photos, or visiting places that were meaningful to both of you can help keep their memory alive and provide solace. Consider opting for professional help in case your grief feels too heavy to bear alone. A counselor or therapist specializing in dealing with grief can provide techniques and tools to take care of your emotions and support you through the entire process.

Avoiding Unhealthy Coping Mechanisms

For some people, grieving may be a long process. It can be tricky to make that transition, and thus, you may develop the wrong ways of handling the situation. In those moments of excessive pain, some will opt to take drugs or alcohol in a bid to dull their feelings. Bereavement has been identified as a cause of substance use disorders, mainly in men (Keyes et al., 2014). It is challenging to grieve when the pain is immense; this means turning to alcohol or drugs can give a brief reprieve but prolongs grief and brings the new difficulty of undoing dependency. Another toxic adjustment technique that many men use is overworking. One of the biggest fears is being alone with your thoughts; hence, when people throw themselves into work, it helps them to avoid their emotions. The key issue with getting busy is that it seems to be nearly helpful in dealing with the grief, although it just hides it. This can make you burn out and take a long time to fully recover that particular aspect of your life.

Another major risk factor is isolation. Isolation is always a dangerous route to take. It is normal to feel like pulling the covers over one's head and telling the incoming days to vanish when one is in pain. However, it is counterproductive to actually do so because the loneliness that sets up camp in the dark may bleak your emotions to make you feel like no one is there for you. The most important thing in loss is to have people around you, and isolating yourself is not healthy at all. It is important not to exhibit such negative ways of dealing with stress, and one must avoid them. On the contrary, learn to process the grief from a healthy perspective since it will help you recover quickly. Some of the possible ways can include speaking with friends, joining support groups of people who also try to seek refuge in isolation, or consultation with a therapist. Taking good care of your health cannot be stressed enough, and this involves taking a balanced diet, getting enough sleep, and abstaining from substances that are poisonous to your body.

Experiencing grief is a process that must not be hurried. And reaching out for a helping hand during this process is to help yourself. In doing so, you will avoid unhealthy ways of coping, and this provides you with the best possibility of recovering from isolating thoughts and tendencies, and grief itself. Do not forget that there is always someone out there to rely on when you catch yourself having thoughts of wanting to isolate yourself.

Overcoming Guilt and Self-Blame

The loss of a relative or a close friend is one of the most painful feelings that a person can experience, but guilt and self-blame typically come right after this. It is likely that one will ruminate over events, questioning if one could have acted in a different way or avoided certain actions. These feelings are natural during the grieving process, but when they come, they can be overwhelming. To overcome such feelings, it is important to come to terms with the fact that this is natural and common. You may not fully understand grief, but what it does to people, especially in relation to guilt or self-blaming scenarios, is that it hinders your ability to be rational and see things objectively. Cognitive-behavioral therapy (CBT) strategies may be particularly useful regarding these thoughts. CBT enables you to dispute and change distorted ways of thinking. For example, if your mind tells you that you could have done more, then change it to: "With the information I had at the time, this is what I could do."

Another effective technique involves practicing forgiveness. Examples include writing an apology letter to yourself for things you might have done wrong or what you think others might not like about you. The fact is, it's okay and acknowledging that you are human is important in order to help address these areas. Psychotherapy can also be of great help. The sudden and acute shift in circumstances can cause a lot of stress, and speaking to a therapist can be very helpful. It's important after any disaster to find someone to talk with and to feel that one can share thoughts and feelings. A psychologist can help one learn how to deal with stress and issues in a constructive way. Telling someone how you feel to a friend or even in a support group can help to lessen the load. It may prove soothing when somebody tells you, "It is not your fault," especially when you are stuck in a difficult situation.

Fear and feeling responsible are elements of the process, but they should not overtake everything. It is important to be patient with yourself and understand that grieving is a complicated process. The process of healing must be liberating, but it does not happen overnight. However, one must learn to cry without feeling like a victim. It is normal to ask for help at any time, and to recognize that you are not the only one going through this.

Breaking Free From Rumination

Rumination can be described as that consistent, frequent reverberation or preoccupation with some past event or even circumstance, where the individual continuously tries to relive the scenario. When grieving, one is stuck in this trap, thinking of what happened, what could have been done to prevent it, or even just thinking of moments spent with the deceased. This cycle just keeps you pinned down; you cannot progress because you keep going back to the memory of pain. Thus, the function of rumination in each type of grief must be comprehended. It can aggravate depression, a sense of guilt, and suicidal intentions. While it is normal to dwell on the loss; however, becoming fixated on these thoughts is not beneficial, and may even be harmful to you.

To free up one's mind from rumination, efforts need to be made deliberately. One of them is to take time each day to look at the future. This is called "worry time". The idea here is to let your mind worry only during this specified time. With this practice, the hold it has over you weakens with time. In case intrusive thoughts happen during other times of the day, tell yourself that they will be addressed during the daily dedicated time set aside for this. One can also get involved in activities that demand concentration as a way of overcoming the problem. There is always beauty in reading a book, doing a crossword puzzle, or even engaging in a hobby, as these can impede negative thoughts. It also means that a walk or any kind of exercise can help change your mind's focus and boost your mood too.

Both mindfulness and grounding are highly effective methods to break this cycle. Mindfulness entails being conscious of the present time, which ultimately helps one to avoid pondering. On the other hand, grounding techniques like paying attention to breathing, the physical feeling of the chair one is sitting on, or focusing on any other object in the surroundings help distract from worrying. Speaking to a therapist can also help to identify with other methods that might be helpful in the given situation for the individual. Professional healthcare workers can assist in changing your negative patterns of thinking and stand by you as you cope with your loss. It is important, and it often takes a lot of time and effort to help a person stop ruminating. As you go through this process, do not be too harsh on yourself. I want to remind you that it is never shameful to get help and to utilize the tools you are given in the healing process.

Combating Chronic Loneliness

Grief is usually followed by loneliness, and thus, one feels enclosed within a cocoon that is very difficult to break through. Even when it comes to seeking help for mental health issues, men are less likely to do so because they may feel it's weak to ask for help. This can lead to a sense of hopelessness, and it may seem like there is no escape from the loneliness that comes with grieving. A particularly effective method in this fight is to dive into new experiential opportunities. Modeling one's regular behavior, or, in other words, attempting something different, be it starting a new leisure activity, practicing a new skill, or just changing your regular route, can be a great way to break the daily routine and create opportunities for interpersonal interaction. These new experiences can lead you to meet like-minded individuals, helping to avoid forced compliance with established social norms and guidelines regarding companionship.

Nature is also something that can have a healing effect when one steps into the green outdoors. It has a way of clearing one's mind and letting one feel at one with Mother Nature - whether it's walking in a park, sitting by a lake, or even discovering new trails. The sounds of nature remind us we are not alone and there is so much more to live for. Another practice that can be followed is to express gratitude. This may initially seem a bit odd, especially when a person is in mourning, but thinking about the positive things in our life changes the focus for a person. It might be useful to write five things you are grateful for in a special notebook every day; this will help you to appreciate what is still available and present.

One may find it fulfilling to adopt a pet, which will offer company and often distractions with their antics. Pets are faithful and capable of enhancing feelings of security that are so important in human lives. Having a pet also increases the chances of getting out of bed to take care of something, which can play a vital role in helping to set a daily routine. Finally, consider professional help. There are several things a therapist can do for loneliness: Gain a voice for your thoughts and feelings, and work on handling your loneliness. There are also other reasons that make therapy useful in dealing with grief, hence helping one to heal. Just remember, everyone feels lonely sometimes, and you are not alone as there are people who can help you. The biggest idea, however, is that there are so many ways to find connection and solace after a loss and taking baby steps can mean big changes in how you will move through your grief.

Chapter 9:
Grief as a Lifelong Journey

Some people see scars, and it is wounding they remember.
To me they are proof of the fact that there is healing.
–Linda Hogan

Grief is a long-term affair, not a one-time phase. It is progressive in that it transforms its form, but rarely does it cease to exist. Grieving is something one learns to live with and needs to find ways of coping with the times when the memories of the deceased may suddenly loom large again. It is not something that you can lock up in the corner and wish for it to disappear the next morning. It can be said that every individual is different, and so is the experience of grieving. There is no correct way to mourn, and there shouldn't be - since grief is deeply personal and differs from one person to another. There are those who will sit and discuss the issue with their friends and families, and there are those who will want to be alone and keep it to themselves. It's crucial to respect your own journey, no matter how it manifests. It's important to note that there is no right or wrong way to grieve, however society may label it or give it a timeline on how one should process it. What you might experience is that the relationship with grief becomes complicated, such that sometimes it can be so invasive, and at other times, it may be more latent.

Why You Will Never "Get Over" Your Loss

One myth that some people often believe is that you should just move on and forget the fact that you lost someone close to you. The loss of a loved one is not something you wake up to the next morning and carry on as if nothing had happened. This is a transformative shift that defines what you are all about. It has been found that continuing bonds with the deceased are theoretically valid, which means it is possible to maintain a close relationship with the person who has died (Stroebe et al., 2010). For instance, I once conversed with a friend, Stephen, who learnt of his father's passing in a rather tragic manner. He narrated how people expected him to get on and carry on with life as if nothing had happened. But for him, his father was present every single day of his life in an abstract form of absence. He stated that simply mentioning his dad, discussing his memories, and even having some of his father's personal items nearby made him feel close. This was not about moving on or getting on with it; it was about learning how to get by and exist with it.

Another man I know, Andrew, who lost his wife due to illness after a long and painful struggle, also said that the pain of losing a loved one is an open sore that never closes. While, over time, its impact may not be as tender and sensitive as a fresh wound, the scar will always be there. By adopting the values that his wife had admired, he was able to pay tribute to her memory and keep her presence in his life. This wasn't progression; rather, it was progressing with grief as a constituent of Andrew's personality. Realizing that you might never recover from the loss makes you more understanding of yourself. Bereavement is not something that happens to people, and then they are done with it. It is a lifelong process in which one must learn to accept the loss as part of life. When you recognize and accept that your connection with the deceased is still present, you allow yourself to mourn at your own pace and style. This approach not only assists you in learning how to survive but also ensures that the love and the memories that you cherish will continue to live with you.

Dealing With Grief Bursts and Sudden Sadness

The intense emotional surges, referred to as grief bursts, occur as minor and random feelings of loss that may come up after several years. These moments can occur at any time. They are usually connected with something: a song that was loved, an aroma, or a place that has been especially dear. They can be rather distressing and confusing, and it makes you realize how much you have lost and that you are still struggling to cope. It is essential to know why grief bursts occur and how they can affect a person. They are natural during bereavement because, again, you retain a connection with the deceased, which is indefinitely continuous. Loss is not a straight-line journey; it is more like a roller coaster ride with several peaks and troughs. However, this stress might commence with time and a particular stimulus that can make you remember your loved one and the relationship you had.

When these moments hit, it's important to acknowledge them rather than push them away. Accept the fact that it is normal to experience jealousy seeing someone else happy when you are grieving. One thing that could be useful is to agree on having a grief ritual—something you do to remind yourself of them every day. This could mean lighting a candle, browsing through family photos, or going for a drive to a place that both of you held close. Another helpful approach is to have a support system in place. This means having friends, relatives, and other competent people who are willing to help if the need arises. For others, merely discussing the feelings can help to reduce the severity of an episode of grief. Such small actions can bring consolation and comfort in the feeling that people are there for you. If you are comfortable with being alone, try putting your thoughts and emotions in writing on a piece of paper or journal. This may assist in reducing feelings of stress and can present you with a better perspective on things.

It is also good to have some kind of coping strategy prepared. Breathe in and out, play some soft music, or take a walk to come back to your senses when you feel that you are stressed. Of course, nobody is perfect, and asking for help from others or seeking help from professional people if needed is alright. These pangs of sorrow are proof of the affection you have and to learn to manage them is a part of growing after the loss.

Finding Joy and Allowing Yourself to Laugh Again

When people are joyful or find themselves laughing after a loss, they may have feelings of guilt. You may ask yourself, "Is it normal to laugh at a time when one is supposed to be sad?" Rest assured that this is normal. The truth is, finding these moments of joy doesn't mean that you are over your loved one or that your grief is any less than anyone else's. It just means that you are an ordinary person with the ability to have feelings. Loss does not mean that you must keep on suffering as a way of paying tribute to the deceased. Nevertheless, it is crucial to understand that grief is not a static experience that remains the same throughout the grieving process. It changes; it is okay to be happy at some point and then be sad at another time. These are times when one should allow themselves to have joyful moments, which is quite normal during the grieving process.

One way to approach this is to think that your loved one would want you to start to find joy again. They would not want your life to be filled with nothing but misery. Happiness and joy are not the betrayal of their memory; they are the embrace of the world's continued beauty. When you accept these happy moments, you are not neglecting or ignoring your love for them, but rather, you are acknowledging the whole of you. If you are still struggling to overcome the guilt, it may help to share your experience with someone who knows what you are going through. Sharing your feelings can help reduce the weight of your sorrow and give you a new outlook on things. It might also be beneficial to establish a particular tradition of remembering the deceased in a manner that enables you to incorporate happiness into the process. It can be as basic as taking a moment to have a laugh in their honor or picturing the smile on their face as they encourage you.

So, it is okay to laugh again. That it is quite all right for you to take pleasure in the things around them. These feelings are proof of your strength and your ability to recover. This does not mean you are over them or forgetting them; it simply means you are going on with your life while they remain in yours.

New Relationships After Loss

It is daunting when one is facing new interpersonal interactions after the loss of a loved one because it is like entering uncharted territory. Indeed, you might find yourself overwhelmed with grief, guilt, and hope all at once. You might be asking if it is too soon, if your feelings are sinful, or if you are cheating on your past. It is worth noting that such feelings are normal and authentic. People should know that forming a new relationship does not require them to forget about the loss of their loved one. Instead, it is a realization that life goes on, and so does the right to love and be happy with whoever the heart chooses. One must learn to allow oneself this phase of life without feeling guilty or overburdened, and it is an important aspect that should be embraced. The heart is versatile enough to accommodate a deeply forgotten past and, at the same time, embrace the future.

In such cases, it is best to engage in effective communication. Do not hide things from your new friend or partner; share how you felt or how things happened. This can help them have the patience and understanding that you need to give them so that they can support your journey. It is also necessary to pay attention to your own emotions and act at a pace that is comfortable for you. In some instances, a new relationship might elicit such feelings as guilt or fear of relapse to the previous station in life. I know many people face this issue, but one must remember that continuing from where one left off is not the same as turning the page completely. It also allows you to remember the one you have lost; at the same time, you can still make new memories. You have a history, and your history has made you the way you are, and these will reflect positively into the new periods in your new relationship.

Thus, to work with such emotions, the primary approach can be to establish a balance between grieving for the past and claiming the future. This could possibly translate to spending some time reviewing your experiences while at the same time creating new ones and connecting with new individuals. It is not easy, yet it is a balancing act, and with time, it is said to become easier. Seek support when needed. You might speak with a therapist or attend group sessions with people in the same boat to share your feelings and get advice on what to do. They present an opportunity to assure an individual that it is possible to experience new relationships again without in any way underemphasizing the importance of the previous relationship.

Relearning Your World as a Griever

Enduring a debilitating loss may permanently change how people interpret events and reality. The process of grieving can lead a person having a different outlook on life, relationships, and self-identity. Loss is a mirror that exposes a person to what is real and ugly about life. In my own experience, I came to learn that everything that I used to take for granted is, in fact, rather vulnerable. The loss has made me pay attention to the fact that life is transient and, at the same time, has made me appreciate life. Suddenly, the daily grind and the everyday errands assumed a new significance. Ordinary things such as admiring a sunset or taking coffee became acts of appreciating the little things in life but also experiences tinged with the melancholy of losing someone dear.

Grief can make the world an alienish place. Activities that were previously enjoyable may now be difficult to find purpose in, or relationships shared with people who have not gone through a loss can feel less fulfilling. This is quite normal since grief is a process that may take some time until the individual reaches the acceptance stage. Your world has changed, and it is okay for you to be disconnected. For many, grieving involves learning how to incorporate this new change into their lives, which can be a difficult process. It is a time-consuming procedure that requires a person to be kind to themselves. It is alright to try to analyze these changes without pruning the process to the shortest possible time. At times, to experience doubt and not be sure of what will happen next, is not unusual.

It is advisable to get in touch with people who have experienced the same kind of loss. People's words and experiences can be soothing in moments of despair and help you realize that you are not alone. Families and friends may not always be understanding or supportive, but other grieving individuals in face-to-face or online support groups can provide that feeling of not being so alone. Grief also helps you develop better empathy and compassion. Despite the loss you have experienced, such deep pain might make you feel more sensitive to others' pain, ready to listen, and help. Gaining this shift can serve as strength and purpose when embarking on the new world. Learning your world over again as a griever is something that we do progressively. It is really about how to acknowledge or continue to mourn the loss while at the same time embracing change in a positive manner. It is important to be patient with oneself during this process. Accept the new situation and understand that it is possible to be happy and have a purpose in the present situation.

The Evolving Seasons of Grief

There is a tendency to describe grief in terms of seasons, meaning that each of them has its peculiarities and transitions. At first, it might be like winter for all that is frosty, bleak, and interminable. This is the kind of response that a person is likely to experience immediately after the loss of a loved one. At some point, temperatures can drop, and one can't help but think that nothing will ever thaw out again. You may be entering a spring of a certain sort as time goes by. This does not mean somehow the pain evaporates, but there is a shift that happens. Gradually, glimmers of hope and revival start to emerge in the otherwise dark universe. This overwhelming despair gradually begins to melt, opening the way for a new kind of civilized dawn.

Grief, as we transit to summertime, is more like a cocktail of warmth and storms. Some days, one gets up and feels that the sun is shining and this brings the opportunity to laugh. And then there are sudden, sharp showers of sadness and longing that catch you when you least anticipate them. Such inconsistency is quite common and natural in the process of mourning. But it is essential to understand that these changes are not a step backward but a natural progression of the process. It might augur that autumn is a time for reflection as well as acceptance. Perhaps the clear and detailed images of the person you lost may offer a certain solace tinged with sadness. This stage is about finding the middle ground between the loss and the incorporation of the lost person into the survivor's life. Sorrow doesn't go away, but it transforms and becomes integrated into the very fiber of one's existence, making life fuller and even more meaningful.

Males are particularly predisposed to experiencing difficulties in mourning due to cultural norms of manliness. Nevertheless, during various seasons of grief, men realize that it is okay to embrace and acknowledge the ability to feel and express emotions as a significant opportunity for growth. Similarly, one could accept this process as a new stage of one's life, accepting the changes of seasons and continuing to cherish the memories of their loved ones.

Helping Others With Your Hard-Won Wisdom

Once you have experienced the storm and the crying of loss, you gather unique knowledge that is very helpful to others. It is a truth born out of suffering, self-reflection, and strength. Passing it on is a way to pay homage to what you have gone through and to help raise hope among those who are just starting their path. In my experience, I have realized that offering help to others with my grief experiences has been both therapeutic and satisfying. It does not mean that my sorrow has vanished or that I possess the final solution, but there is comfort in knowing that, together with the person, I can trace the pain. Let us assume there is a friend who has recently gone through the painful experience of burying a close relative. They are still in the first and most chaotic stage of grief and despair. With that, you may be able to explain some of the things that they are feeling based on your own experiences. You can let them know that it is alright to mourn as they wish and that there are no rules that anyone has to adhere to. Such support can be truly beneficial.

There is also authority in silence and having an ear to listen. Often, what is required is not giving advice but giving someone a platform to pour out their suffering. It is about being there for them and letting them shout, cry, or even just sit in moments of silence. Your mere presence can be a beacon in their stormy sea. Research has revealed that support from peers can go a long way in helping with grief (Bartone et al., 2017). Speaking to a person who has undergone a similar experience can help you cope effectively with loneliness and find some hope. Your story, your insights, and your compassion may be literally lifesaving for someone else. Consider volunteering for grief support groups and becoming a grief support group leader or mentor. Your experiences make you better placed to give advice and offer words of encouragement. You can also share coping strategies that helped you or simply just be an example of how life goes on.

It is also important to note that assisting others in going through their grief also serves the dual purpose of strengthening the individual's own recovery. It forms a cycle of compassion by showing that even in the horrific place of despair, there is hope and a bond to be found. The journey through grief is a chance to offer hope to those who walk the same path and to turn pain into help.

Chapter 10:
Honoring Your Journey

Grief, I've learned, is really just love. It's all the love you want to give but cannot.
–Jamie Anderson

Navigating through the previous chapters, you have been introduced to the multiple sides of grief and how it pervades every aspect of an individual's life. This means, of course, that we have talked about the challenges as well as the possible ways one can manage them, all the while bearing in mind that grieving is a very individual process. It is also necessary to accept and celebrate one's journey during this process to understand that it is fine and necessary to have such feelings. The concept of this chapter is to let yourself mourn, and to mourn in the way that you want to. It's about acknowledging that the feelings you have—positive and negative, rational and irrational—are entirely normal in the face of loss. This means acknowledging that you value your entire story, and that you have room for the process of overcoming challenges. In this section, we will discuss the necessity of having self-compassion and validation, the importance of reminding yourself that it is alright to grieve, and that your feelings are essential in the healing process.

Understanding Your Grief Journey

It is crucial that you learn more about the process you are going through as you make your way through this difficult time. Bereavement is a complex process that can be quite different in each case, depending on the individual. The grieving process includes everything you think, feel, or do while coming to terms with the loss of a person. It is also crucial to understand that grief does not have an ideal model and cannot be accompanied by any specific time frame. The theory proposed by Kübler-Ross is based on the five stages of grieving, namely denial, anger, bargaining, depression, and finally, acceptance (Rogers, 2022). While these stages might help to identify some of the feelings one would expect, one must keep in mind that these stages are not sequential. It can be noted that you may go through each stage for some time; some stages you may not go through at all; or you may go through the stages in a different order. Such inconsistency is understandable within this process.

Everyone grieves in a different way based on the relationship they had with the deceased, his personality, culture, and history of losses. What is consistent across cultures, though, is the ability to let yourself cry and to process those feelings. The inability to acknowledge or listen to your emotions can greatly slow or even prevent the healing process. Therefore, when you accept your individuality and allow yourself to mourn in your own manner, it is possible to progress toward positive change. It is important to know that your feelings of grief are natural, and there is no fixed way of grieving.

Acceptance and Acknowledgement

It is incredibly important that you accept and embrace your emotions in order to start the healing process. Most people experience emotions of all types after loss, and it is okay to feel sad, angry, confused, and relieved in some ways. These feelings may be so intense that one might feel the need to reject or ignore them, especially when people around you, your friends and family, just want you to be "strong" and "carry on". Embracing and feeling these emotions are necessary to heal genuinely. It is important to let out your feelings, as repressing them has long-term psychological and bodily effects. This might appear to be a "temporary fix" or a "denial of grief", but unlabeled grief can cause harm in the long run, impacting one's physical and psychological well-being. However, when you acknowledge these feelings, it does not necessarily mean that you must approve of them or even appreciate them. It is as simple as acknowledging their presence and allowing yourself to experience them.

It is a major step towards healing when you recognize that you do indeed have pain. It lets you accept the reality of the loss and work it through into your life. This does not mean the pain will go away, but it can be somewhat tolerable. If you confront this, then you are able to deal with the pain in a constructive manner. This can often be a challenging process, but it is a critical step in a person's journey to establishing a new routine. Always bear in mind, though, that all your emotions, however complex, are real and genuine. You must respect them, embrace them, and let the soul heal as it undergoes the process of grieving and coping. It is alright to feel the pain, and it is equally alright to take your time feeling the pain. Forgetting can be an impossibility of healing, nor its intention; it is all about coming to terms with the loss while acknowledging the death of the loved one.

Honoring Your Loved One and Yourself

Honoring your special someone is a beneficial component of mourning and a significant way to pay tribute to him or her. For instance, creating a memory box at home might be helpful to hold all the sweet memories you had with your loved one. The box could be adorned with pictures, letters, and other tokens that you would like to capture the times you were with your loved one. Having this tangible collection of memories can be somewhat soothing since it constantly reminds the individual of the love and joy they brought to our life. It is also possible to write letters to your beloved as this can also be a good expressive exercise while writing down thoughts and emotions. This action can make us feel connected to them and can be carried out as a daily or weekly practice, or whatever frequency feels apt. These letters can serve as an outlet for the emotional self, where one can weep and talk about daily life, grief, or happy moments.

Alternatively, a tree can be planted in their honor to represent a new beginning or symbolize a new chapter after the passing. Watching the tree grow over the years can be an example of a living memorial to the person who has influenced your life. This is a lovely method of honoring them and making certain the spirit of their lives is captured with the seasons of nature. Honoring your loved one may be useful when grieving because it offers a specific way to deal with the feelings of loss. It provides you with the feeling that you are not alone, that others have also experienced what you have, and it assists you in incorporating the loss into your life story. All these actions let you keep your loved one alive in your mind and heart and are therefore comforting and healing.

Equally important is taking care of oneself during this period. Grief takes a toll on your physical and mental health, and therefore, you need to take proper care of yourself. Take care of your body by eating healthy, exercising, and following a proper sleep cycle. These are simple needs that may be easily ignored during times of grief, but they are highly important for your health. Self-care involves physical health, and mental health is as essential as physical health. Confiding in friends, relatives, or even a professional counselor is very helpful in providing comfort and direction. Sharing your emotions with someone also assists in overcoming the depressive state and feelings of loneliness due to the loss. If there is something that you consider difficult, then it is okay to seek assistance, as nobody is flawless.

Be gentle with yourself and move forward at your own pace. You have a lot left in life.

Conclusion

As we come to the end of this journey together, I want you to know that I truly understand the unique and often unspoken grief that men endure. Grieving is never a linear process, and as men, there is always this culturally imposed burden of having to bear the pain and maintain a stiff upper lip. However, your grief is real, and your emotions should not be silenced or suppressed. Throughout this book, I have tried to explain numerous facets of grief and how they impact men. Ranging from social pressure and expectations to the inner struggles associated with bereavement, every chapter is intended to introduce the reader to the shades of grey of your story. One should know that there is no specific approach - no right or wrong way - regarding how to grieve. Remember that everyone's path is unique and that it is perfectly acceptable for you to traverse this journey at your own speed.

Grieving can change the way one relates to others, modify one's identity, and even revolutionize one's perception of the world. It is very subjective and often results in loneliness and feelings of non-recognition. But remember, you are not the only one grieving. Unfortunately, it is very common. Many men have been in this position, and there are ways to care for your loved ones without neglecting yourself. I truly hope that the strategies and stories presented in this book have provided you with some solace and useful guidance. Whether it is letting yourself cry, going to a professional, or making a memory box - that is progress toward healing. It is not impossible or even wrong to honor the memory of your loved one while also not neglecting yourself.

Grief over loss does not linger for a period but lasts for a lifetime, and thus, people, especially men, should learn how to embrace it. It becomes an integral aspect of yourself and one that changes you in ways you perhaps could not anticipate. Take everything with grace; accept that life is a roller coaster of emotions; and understand that it is okay to be happy and sad simultaneously. May you find comfort, courage, and wisdom in the process you are going through in relation to your loss. Remember, it is perfectly alright to ask for help, seek support, and cherish your loved one and yourself in a loving manner. Your path is significant, and you are allowed to have such emotions. Stay well, and don't be too harsh on yourself.

A Note From the Author

It is ironic that just as I was finishing writing this book, my father (unawares of my writings) shared about how he held himself together when he heard of his father's death. It was only when he made the journey back to his hometown and saw his mother, that he could cry uncontrollably in her arms. My heart went out to him when I heard him telling us this – only now when he is a grandfather. I am glad he had a safe space to grief eventually, and no man should feel lacking such a basic need.

This book is for him, and men like him, to know that it is important to cry, to speak, to feel, to understand, to embrace, and to heal. The grief of men must be spoken about.

Thank you for including **The Unspoken Grief of Men** in your healing journey. I hope you found it useful and will share this companion guide with other men who may also benefit from it. Your review will benefit others also going through a painful time of loss.

You can leave your thoughts and comments at

https://www.amazon.com/dp/B0DCT24J1M

Yours sincerely,

SL Hans

References

Bartone, P. T., Bartone, J. V., Violanti, J. M., & Gileno, Z. M. (2017). Peer support services for bereaved survivors: A systematic review. *OMEGA - Journal of Death and Dying*, *80*(1), 137–166. https://doi.org/10.1177/0030222817728204

Chaplin, T. M. (2018). Gender and emotion expression: A developmental contextual perspective. *Emotion Review*, *7*(1), 14–21. https://doi.org/10.1177/1754073914544408

Disenfranchised grief. (2023, August 15). Wikipedia. https://en.wikipedia.org/wiki/Disenfranchised_grief

Doka, K. J. (1999). Disenfranchised grief. Bereavement Care, 18(3), 37–39. https://doi.org/10.1080/02682629908657467

Grief, bereavement, and coping with loss. (2017). National Cancer Institute; Cancer.gov. https://www.cancer.gov/about-cancer/advanced-cancer/caregivers/planning/bereavement-hp-pdq

Gross, J. J., Fredrickson, B. L., & Levenson, R. W. (1994). The psychophysiology of crying. *Psychophysiology*, *31*(5), 460–468. https://doi.org/10.1111/j.1469-8986.1994.tb01049.x

Hewson, H., Galbraith, N., Jones, C., & Heath, G. (2023). The impact of continuing bonds following bereavement. *Death Studies*, 1–14. https://doi.org/10.1080/07481187.2023.2223593

Hogan, N. S., Schmidt, L. A., Howard Sharp, K. M., Barrera, M., Compas, B. E., Davies, B., Fairclough, D. L., Gilmer, M. J., Vannatta, K., & Gerhardt, C. A. (2019). Development and testing of the Hogan Inventory of Bereavement short form for children and adolescents. *Death Studies*, 1–9. https://doi.org/10.1080/07481187.2019.1627034

Hurrying Through Grief: Returning to work after a death. (n.d.). Www.linkedin.com. Retrieved June 3, 2024, from https://www.linkedin.com/pulse/hurrying-through-grief-returning-work-after-death-darin-d-/

John Green quote. (n.d.). A-Z Quotes. Retrieved June 4, 2024, from https://www.azquotes.com/quote/1390370

Keyes, K. M., Pratt, C., Galea, S., McLaughlin, K. A., Koenen, K. C., & Shear, M. K. (2014). The burden of loss: Unexpected death of a loved one and psychiatric disorders across the life course in a national study. *American Journal of Psychiatry*, *171*(8), 864–871. https://doi.org/10.1176/appi.ajp.2014.13081132

Klass, D. (2006). Continuing conversation about continuing bonds. *Death Studies*, *30*(9), 843–858. https://doi.org/10.1080/07481180600886959

Mancini, A. D., & Bonanno, G. A. (2009). Predictors and parameters of resilience to loss: Toward an individual differences model. *Journal of Personality*, *77*(6), 1805–1832. https://doi.org/10.1111/j.1467-6494.2009.00601.x

Neimeyer, R. (2005). Grief, loss, and the quest for meaning. *Bereavement Care*, *24*(2), 27–30. https://doi.org/10.1080/02682620508657628

Pederson, E. L., & Vogel, D. L. (2007). Male gender role conflict and willingness to seek counseling: *Journal of Counseling Psychology*, *54*(4), 373–384. https://doi.org/10.1037/0022-0167.54.4.373

Pk, M., B, Z., Sd, B., & Hg, P. (2007, February 21). *An empirical examination of the stage theory of grief.* JAMA. https://pubmed.ncbi.nlm.nih.gov/17312291/

Queen   Elizabeth   II   quotes.   (n.d.).   BrainyQuote.
    https://www.brainyquote.com/quotes/queen_elizabeth_ii_178
    865

Quote   by   Alphonse   de   Lamartine.   (n.d.).
    https://www.brainyquote.com/quotes/alphonse_de_lamartine
    _143018

Quote   by   Anne   Lamott.   (n.d.).   Www.goodreads.com.
    https://www.goodreads.com/quotes/70759-you-will-lose-
    someone-you-can-t-live-without-and-your-heart

Quote   by   Jamie   Anderson.   (n.d.).   Www.goodreads.com.
    https://www.goodreads.com/quotes/9657488-grief-i-ve-
    learned-is-really-just-love-it-s-all-the

Quote by Kahlil Gibran. (n.d.). Www.goodreads.com. Retrieved June 6,
    2024,   from   https://www.goodreads.com/quotes/767-when-
    you-are-sorrowful-look-again-in-your-heart-and

Quote by Kenji Miyazawa. (n.d.). Www.goodreads.com. Retrieved June 6,
    2024,   from   https://www.goodreads.com/quotes/35468-we-
    must-embrace-pain-and-burn-it-as-fuel-for

Quote   by   Leo   Tolstoy.   (n.d.).   Www.goodreads.com.
    https://www.goodreads.com/quotes/36797-only-people-who-
    are-capable-of-loving-strongly-can-also

Quote   by   Linda   Hogan.   (n.d.).   Www.goodreads.com.
    https://www.goodreads.com/quotes/259422-some-people-
    see-scars-and-it-is-wounding-they-remember

Quote   by   Vicki   Harrison.   (n.d.).   Www.goodreads.com.
    https://www.goodreads.com/quotes/543175-grief-is-like-the-
    ocean-it-comes-on-waves-ebbing

Quote from A Grief Observed. (n.d.). Www.goodreads.com. Retrieved May 31, 2024, from https://www.goodreads.com/quotes/707905-grief-is-like-a-long-valley-a-winding-valley-where

Quote from The Return of the King. (n.d.). Www.goodreads.com. Retrieved May 29, 2024, from https://www.goodreads.com/quotes/37414-i-will-not-say-do-not-weep-for-not-all

Rogers, K. (2022, July 28). *5 stages of grief, and how to get through them.* CNN. https://edition.cnn.com/2021/09/12/health/five-stages-of-grief-kubler-ross-meaning-wellness/index.html

Role of rituals in the grieving process. (n.d.). https://www.internationalcollegeofprofessionalcelebrants.org/blog/the-role-of-rituals-in-the-grieving-process

Ruan, Y., Reis, H. T., Zareba, W., & Lane, R. D. (2019). Does suppressing negative emotion impair subsequent emotions? *Motivation and Emotion.* https://doi.org/10.1007/s11031-019-09774-w

Shear, K., Frank, E., Houck, P. R., & Reynolds, C. F. (2005). Treatment of complicated grief. *JAMA, 293*(21), 2601. https://doi.org/10.1001/jama.293.21.2601

Stroebe, M., & Schut, H. (1999). The dual process model of coping with bereavement: Rationale and description. *Death Studies, 23*(3), 197–224. https://doi.org/10.1080/074811899201046

Stroebe, M., Schut, H., & Boerner, K. (2010). Continuing bonds in adaptation to bereavement. *Clinical Psychology Review, 30*(2), 259–268. https://doi.org/10.1016/j.cpr.2009.11.007

Understanding different grieving patterns in your family. (2017). https://hov.org/media/1765/bit-jul-aug-2017.pdf

Utz, R. L., Caserta, M., & Lund, D. (2011). Grief, depressive symptoms, and physical health among recently bereaved spouses. *The Gerontologist,* *52*(4), 460–471. https://doi.org/10.1093/geront/gnr110

When someone you love becomes a memory quote. (n.d.). AllAuthor. https://allauthor.com/quotes/12252/

Wolf, C. C. (2024, February 27). *How the brain copes with grief.* Scientific American. https://www.scientificamerican.com/article/how-the-brain-copes-with-grief/

Zoellner, T., & Maercker, A. (2006). Posttraumatic growth in clinical psychology — A critical review and introduction of a two component model. *Clinical Psychology Review, 26*(5), 626–653. https://doi.org/10.1016/j.cpr.2006.01.008

Made in the USA
Las Vegas, NV
08 January 2025

16077262R00061